Virtual Clinical Excursions—Medical-Surgical

for

Cooper and Gosnell:
Adult Health Nursing
7th Edition

Virtual Clinical Excursions—Medical-Surgical

for

Cooper and Gosnell:
Adult Health Nursing
7th Edition

prepared by

Kim D. Cooper, RN, MSN
Dean, School of Nursing
Ivy Tech Community College
Terre Haute, Indiana

software developed by

Wolfsong Informatics, LLC
Tucson, Arizona

ELSEVIER
MOSBY

ELSEVIER
MOSBY

3251 Riverport Lane
Maryland Heights, Missouri 63043

VIRTUAL CLINICAL EXCURSIONS—MEDICAL-SURGICAL FOR
COOPER AND GOSNELL:
ADULT HEALTH NURSING
SEVENTH EDITION

ISBN: 978-0-323-22179-5

Copyright © 2015 by Mosby, an imprint of Elsevier Inc.
Copyright © 2011, 2007 by Mosby, Inc., an affiliate of Elsevier Inc.

ISBN: 978-0-323-22179-5

Printed in the United States of America

Last digit is the print number: 9 8 7 6 5 4 3 2 1

Workbook
prepared by

Kim D. Cooper, RN, MSN
Dean, School of Nursing
Ivy Tech Community College
Terre Haute, Indiana

Textbook

Kim Cooper, RN, MSN
Dean, School of Nursing
Ivy Tech Community College
Terre Haute, Indiana

Kelly Gosnell, RN, MSN
Associate Professor
School of Nursing
Ivy Tech Community College
Terre Haute, Indiana

Table of Contents
Virtual Clinical Excursions Workbook

Getting Started

Getting Set Up with VCE Online 1
A Quick Tour 3
A Detailed Tour 19
Reducing Medication Errors 31

Unit 1—Care of the Patient with a Musculoskeletal Disorder

Lesson 1   Assessment of the Patient with Osteomyelitis (Chapters 3 and 4) 37
Lesson 2   Care of the Patient Experiencing Comorbid Conditions
           (Musculoskeletal and Endocrine) (Chapter 11) 47
Lesson 3   Developing a Plan of Care for the Patient with Osteomyelitis (Chapter 4) . . . 55

Unit 2—Care of the Surgical Patient

Lesson 4   Postoperative Assessment (Chapters 2 and 4) 61
Lesson 5   Postoperative Complications (Chapters 2 and 9) 69

Unit 3—Care of the Patient with a Respiratory Disorder

Lesson 6   Care of the Patient with Pneumonia (Chapter 9) 79
Lesson 7   Care of the Patient Experiencing Comorbid Conditions
           (Musculoskeletal and Respiratory) (Chapters 4, 8, and 9) 87
Lesson 8   Prioritizing Care for the Patient with a Pulmonary Disorder (Chapter 9) 95

Unit 4—Care of the Patient with Asthma

Lesson 9   Care of the Patient Experiencing Exacerbation of an Asthmatic Condition
           (Chapter 9) 103
Lesson 10 Developing a Plan of Care for the Asthmatic Patient with
           Psychological Complications (Chapter 9) 111

Unit 5—Care of the Patient Diagnosed with Cancer

Lesson 11 Care and Treatment of the Patient with Complications of Cancer
           (Chapter 17) 119
Lesson 12 Care and Treatment of the Patient with Cancer (Chapter 17) 129

Unit 6—Care of the Patient with a Gastrointestinal Disorder

Lesson 13 Assessment of the Patient with Gastrointestinal Complications (Chapter 5) . . 137
Lesson 14 Colorectal Cancer and Care of the Patient After Gastrointestinal Surgery
           (Chapters 2 and 5) 147

Table of Contents
Cooper and Gosnell:
Adult Health Nursing, 7th Edition

Chapter 1   Introduction to Anatomy and Physiology

Chapter 2   Care of the Surgical Patient (Lessons 4, 5, and 14)

Chapter 3   Care of the Patient with an Integumentary Disorder (Lesson 1)

Chapter 4   Care of the Patient with a Musculoskeletal Disorder (Lessons 1, 3, 4, and 7)

Chapter 5   Care of the Patient with a Gastrointestinal Disorder (Lessons 13 and 14)

Chapter 6   Care of the Patient with a Gallbladder, Liver, Biliary Tract, or Exocrine Pancreatic Disorder

Chapter 7   Care of the Patient with a Blood or Lymphatic Disorder

Chapter 8   Care of the Patient with a Cardiovascular or a Peripheral Vascular Disorder (Lesson 7)

Chapter 9   Care of the Patient with a Respiratory Disorder (Lessons 5, 6, 7, 8, 9, and 10)

Chapter 10 Care of the Patient with a Urinary Disorder

Chapter 11 Care of the Patient with an Endocrine Disorder (Lesson 2)

Chapter 12 Care of the Patient with a Reproductive Disorder

Chapter 13 Care of the Patient with a Visual or Auditory Disorder

Chapter 14 Care of the Patient with a Neurologic Disorder

Chapter 15 Care of the Patient with an Immune Disorder

Chapter 16 Care of the Patient with HIV/AIDS

Chapter 17 Care of the Patient with Cancer (Lessons 11 and 12)

GETTING SET UP WITH VCE ONLINE

The product you have purchased is part of the Evolve Learning System. Please read the following information thoroughly to get started.

■ HOW TO ACCESS YOUR VCE RESOURCES ON EVOLVE

There are two ways to access your VCE Resources on Evolve:

1. If your instructor has enrolled you in your VCE Evolve Resources, you will receive an email with your registration details.

2. If your instructor has asked you to self-enroll in your VCE Evolve Resources, he or she will provide you with your Course ID (for example, 1479_jdoe73_0001). You will then need to follow the instructions at https://evolve.elsevier.com/cs/studentEnroll.html.

■ HOW TO ACCESS THE ONLINE VIRTUAL HOSPITAL

The online virtual hospital is available through the Evolve VCE Resources. There is no software to download or install: the online virtual hospital runs within your Internet browser, using a pop-up window.

■ TECHNICAL REQUIREMENTS

- Broadband connection (DSL or cable)
- 1024 x 768 screen resolution
- Mozilla Firefox 18.0, Internet Explorer 9.0, Google Chrome, or Safari 5 (or higher)
  Note: Pop-up blocking software/settings must be disabled.
- Adobe Acrobat Reader
- Additional technical requirements available at http://evolvesupport.elsevier.com

■ HOW TO ACCESS THE WORKBOOK

There are two ways to access the workbook portion of *Virtual Clinical Excursions:*

1. Print workbook
2. An electronic version of the workbook, available within the VCE Evolve Resources

■ TECHNICAL SUPPORT

Technical support for *Virtual Clinical Excursions* is available by visiting the Technical Support Center at http://evolvesupport.elsevier.com or by calling 1-800-222-9570 inside the United States and Canada.

Trademarks: Windows® and Macintosh® are registered trademarks.

A QUICK TOUR

Welcome to *Virtual Clinical Excursions—Medical-Surgical*, a virtual hospital setting in which you can work with multiple complex patient simulations and also learn to access and evaluate the information resources that are essential for high-quality patient care. The virtual hospital, Pacific View Regional Hospital, has realistic architecture and access to patient rooms, a Nurses' Station, and a Medication Room.

■ BEFORE YOU START

Make sure you have your textbook nearby when you use *Virtual Clinical Excursions*. You will want to consult topic areas in your textbook frequently while working with the virtual hospital and workbook.

■ HOW TO SIGN IN

- Enter your name on the Student Nurse identification badge.
- Now choose one of the four periods of care in which to work. In Periods of Care 1 through 3, you can actively engage in patient assessment, entry of data in the electronic patient record (EPR), and medication administration. Period of Care 4 presents the day in review. Highlight and click the appropriate period of care. (For this quick tour, choose **Period of Care 1: 0730-0815**.)
- This takes you to the Patient List screen (see the *How to Select a Patient* section below). Only the patients on the Medical-Surgical Floor are available. Note that the virtual time is provided in the box at the lower left corner of the screen (0730, since we chose Period of Care 1).

Note: If you choose to work during Period of Care 4: 1900-2000, the Patient List screen is skipped since you are not able to visit patients or administer medications during the shift. Instead, you are taken directly to the Nurses' Station, where the records of all the patients on the floor are available for your review.

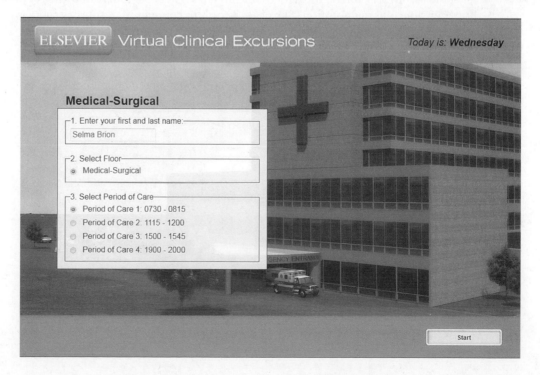

■ PATIENT LIST

MEDICAL-SURGICAL UNIT

Harry George (Room 401)
Osteomyelitis—A 54-year-old Caucasian male admitted from a homeless shelter with an infected leg. He has complications of type 2 diabetes mellitus, alcohol abuse, nicotine addiction, poor pain control, and complex psychosocial issues.

Jacquline Catanazaro (Room 402)
Asthma—A 45-year-old Caucasian female admitted with an acute asthma exacerbation and suspected pneumonia. She has complications of chronic schizophrenia, noncompliance with medication therapy, obesity, and herniated disc.

Piya Jordan (Room 403)
Bowel obstruction—A 68-year-old Asian female admitted with a colon mass and suspected adenocarcinoma. She undergoes a right hemicolectomy. This patient's complications include atrial fibrillation, hypokalemia, and symptoms of meperidine toxicity.

Clarence Hughes (Room 404)
Degenerative joint disease—A 73-year-old African-American male admitted for a left total knee replacement. His preparations for discharge are complicated by the development of a pulmonary embolus and the need for ongoing intravenous therapy.

Pablo Rodriguez (Room 405)
Metastatic lung carcinoma—A 71-year-old Hispanic male admitted with symptoms of dehydration and malnutrition. He has chronic pain secondary to multiple subcutaneous skin nodules and psychosocial concerns related to family issues with his approaching death.

Patricia Newman (Room 406)
Pneumonia—A 61-year-old Caucasian female admitted with worsening pulmonary function and an acute respiratory infection. Her chronic emphysema is complicated by heavy smoking, hypertension, and malnutrition. She needs access to community resources such as a smoking cessation program and meal assistance.

■ HOW TO SELECT A PATIENT

- You can choose one or more patients to work with from the Patient List by checking the box to the left of the patient name(s). For this quick tour, select Piya Jordan and Pablo Rodriguez. (In order to receive a scorecard for a patient, the patient must be selected before proceeding to the Nurses' Station.)
- Click on **Get Report** to the right of the medical records number (MRN) to view a summary of the patient's care during the 12-hour period before your arrival on the unit.
- After reviewing the report, click on **Go to Nurses' Station** in the right lower corner to begin your care. (*Note:* If you have been assigned to care for multiple patients, you can click on **Return to Patient List** to select and review the report for each additional patient before going to the Nurses' Station.)

Note: Even though the Patient List is initially skipped when you sign in to work for Period of Care 4, you can still access this screen if you wish to review the shift report for any of the patients. To do so, simply click on **Patient List** near the top left corner of the Nurses' Station (or click on the clipboard to the left of the Kardex). Then click on **Get Report** for the patient(s) whose care you are reviewing. This may be done during any period of care.

Patient List

	Patient Name	Room	MRN	Clinical Report
☐	Harry George	401	1868054	Get Report
☐	Jacquline Catanazaro	402	1868048	Get Report
☑	Piya Jordan	403	1868092	Get Report
☐	Clarence Hughes	404	1868011	Get Report
☑	Pablo Rodriguez	405	1868088	Get Report
☐	Patricia Newman	406	1868097	Get Report

Please select all the patients you will be caring for this period of care. Once you have exited the patient list, you will not be able to change your current selections or select new patients to care for.

0730   Go to Nurses' Station

■ HOW TO FIND A PATIENT'S RECORDS

NURSES' STATION

Within the Nurses' Station, you will see:

1. A clipboard that contains the patient list for that floor.
2. A chart rack with patient charts labeled by room number, a notebook labeled Kardex, and a notebook labeled MAR (Medication Administration Record).
3. A desktop computer with access to the Electronic Patient Record (EPR).
4. A tool bar across the top of the screen that can also be used to access the Patient List, EPR, Chart, MAR, and Kardex. This tool bar is also accessible from each patient's room.
5. A Drug Guide containing information about the medications you are able to administer to your patients.
6. A Laboratory Guide containing normal value ranges for all laboratory tests you may come across in the virtual patient hospital.
7. A tool bar across the bottom of the screen that can be used to access the Floor Map, patient rooms, Medication Room, and Drug Guide.

As you run your cursor over an item, it will be highlighted. To select, simply click on the item. As you use these resources, you will always be able to return to the Nurses' Station by clicking on the **Return to Nurses' Station** bar located in the right lower corner of your screen.

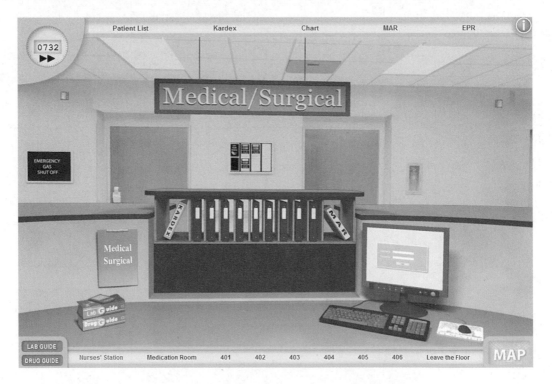

MEDICATION ADMINISTRATION RECORD (MAR)

The MAR icon located on the tool bar at the top of your screen accesses current 24-hour medications for each patient. Click on the icon and the MAR will open. (*Note:* You can also access the MAR by clicking on the MAR notebook on the far right side of the book rack in the center of the screen.) Within the MAR, tabs on the right side of the screen allow you to select patients by room number. Be careful to make sure you select the correct tab number for *your* patient rather than simply reading the first record that appears after the MAR opens. Each MAR sheet lists the following:

- Medications
- Route and dosage of each medication
- Times of administration of each medication

Note: The MAR changes each day. Expired MARs are stored in the patients' charts.

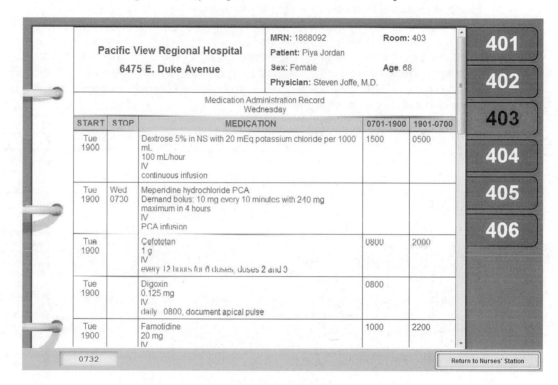

CHARTS

To access patient charts, either click on the **Chart** icon at the top of your screen or anywhere within the chart rack in the center of the Nurses' Station screen. When the close-up view appears, the individual charts are labeled by room number. To open a chart, click on the room number of the patient whose chart you wish to review. The patient's name and allergies will appear on the left side of the screen, along with a list of tabs on the right side of the screen, allowing you to view the following data:

- Allergies
- Physician's Orders
- Physician's Notes
- Nurse's Notes
- Laboratory Reports
- Diagnostic Reports
- Surgical Reports
- Consultations

- Patient Education
- History and Physical
- Nursing Admission
- Expired MARs
- Consents
- Mental Health
- Admissions
- Emergency Department

Information appears in real time. The entries are in reverse chronologic order, so use the down arrow at the right side of each chart page to scroll down to view previous entries. Flip from tab to tab to view multiple data fields or click on **Return to Nurses' Station** in the lower right corner of the screen to exit the chart.

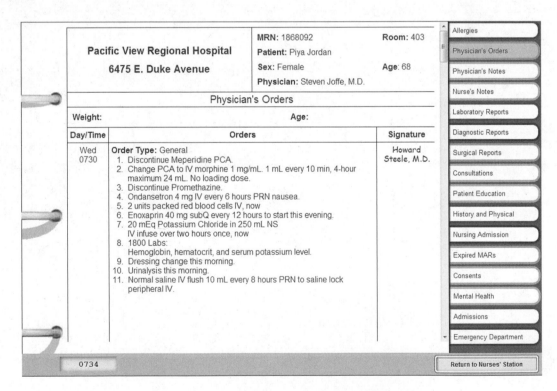

ELECTRONIC PATIENT RECORD (EPR)

The EPR can be accessed from the computer in the Nurses' Station or from the EPR icon located in the tool bar at the top of your screen. To access a patient's EPR:
- Click on either the computer screen or the **EPR** icon.
- Your username and password are automatically filled in.
- Click on **Login** to enter the EPR.
- *Note:* Like the MAR, the EPR is arranged numerically. Thus when you enter, you are initially shown the records of the patient in the lowest room number on the floor. To view the correct data for *your* patient, remember to select the correct room number, using the drop-down menu for the Patient field at the top left corner of the screen.

The EPR used in Pacific View Regional Hospital represents a composite of commercial versions being used in hospitals. You can access the EPR:
- to review existing data for a patient (by room number).
- to enter data you collect while working with a patient.

The EPR is updated daily, so no matter what day or part of a shift you are working, there will be a current EPR with the patient's data from the past days of the current hospital stay. This type of simulated EPR allows you to examine how data for different attributes have changed over time, as well as to examine data for all of a patient's attributes at a particular time. The EPR is fully functional (as it is in a real-life hospital). You can enter such data as blood pressure, breath sounds, and certain treatments. The EPR will not, however, allow you to enter data for a previous time period. Use the arrows at the bottom of the screen to move forward and backward in time.

Patient: 403	Category: Vital Signs			0735	
Name: Piya Jordan	Wed 0630	Wed 0700	Wed 0715	Code Meanings	
PAIN: LOCATION		OS		A	Abdomen
PAIN: RATING		5		Ar	Arm
PAIN: CHARACTERISTICS		C		B	Back
PAIN: VOCAL CUES		VC3		C	Chest
PAIN: FACIAL CUES		FC1		Ft	Foot
PAIN: BODILY CUES				H	Head
PAIN: SYSTEM CUES				Hd	Hand
PAIN: FUNCTIONAL EFFECTS				L	Left
PAIN: PREDISPOSING FACTORS				Lg	Leg
PAIN: RELIEVING FACTORS				Lw	Lower
PCA		P		N	Neck
TEMPERATURE (F)		99.6		NN	See Nurses notes
TEMPERATURE (C)				OS	Operative site
MODE OF MEASUREMENT		Ty		Or	See Physicians orders
SYSTOLIC PRESSURE		110		PN	See Progress notes
DIASTOLIC PRESSURE		70		R	Right
BP MODE OF MEASUREMENT		NIBP		Up	Upper
HEART RATE		104			
RESPIRATORY RATE		18			
SpO2 (%)		95			
BLOOD GLUCOSE					
WEIGHT					
HEIGHT					

Return to Nurses' Station

At the top of the EPR screen, you can choose patients by their room numbers. In addition, you have access to 17 different categories of patient data. To change patients or data categories, click the down arrow to the right of the room number or category.

The categories of patient data in the EPR are as follows:

- Vital Signs
- Respiratory
- Cardiovascular
- Neurologic
- Gastrointestinal
- Excretory
- Musculoskeletal
- Integumentary
- Reproductive
- Psychosocial
- Wounds and Drains
- Activity
- Hygiene and Comfort
- Safety
- Nutrition
- IV
- Intake and Output

Remember, each hospital selects its own codes. The codes used in the EPR at Pacific View Regional Hospital may be different from ones you have seen in your clinical rotations. Take some time to acquaint yourself with the codes. Within the Vital Signs category, click on any item in the left column (e.g., Pain: Characteristics). In the far-right column, you will see a list of code meanings for the possible findings and/or descriptors for that assessment area.

You will use the codes to record the data you collect as you work with patients. Click on the box in the last time column to the right of any item and wait for the code meanings applicable to that entry to appear. Select the appropriate code to describe your assessment findings and type it in the box. (*Note:* If no cursor appears within the box, click on the box again until the blue shading disappears and the blinking cursor appears.) Once the data are typed in this box, they are entered into the patient's record for this period of care only.

To leave the EPR, click on **Exit EPR** in the bottom right corner of the screen.

■ VISITING A PATIENT

From the Nurses' Station, click on the room number of the patient you wish to visit (in the tool bar at the bottom of your screen). Once you are inside the room, you will see a still photo of your patient in the top left corner. To verify that this is the correct patient, click on the **Check Armband** icon to the right of the photo. The patient's identification data will appear. If you click on **Check Allergies** (the next icon to the right), a list of the patient's allergies (if any) will replace the photo.

Also located in the patient's room are multiple icons you can use to assess the patient or the patient's medications. A virtual clock is provided in the upper left corner of the room to monitor your progress in real time. (*Note:* The fast-forward icon within the virtual clock will advance the time by 2-minute intervals when clicked.)

- The tool bar across the top of the screen allows you to check the **Patient List**, access the **EPR** to check or enter data, and view the patient's **Chart**, **MAR**, or **Kardex**.

- The **Take Vital Signs** icon allows you to measure the patient's up-to-the-minute blood pressure, oxygen saturation, temperature, heart rate, respiratory rate, and pain level.

- Each time you enter a patient's room, you are given an Initial Observation report to review (in the text box under the patient's photo). These notes are provided to give you a "look" at the patient as if you had just stepped into the room. You can also click on the **Initial Observations** icon to return to this box from other views within the patient's room. To the right of this icon is **Clinical Alerts**, a resource that allows you to make decisions about priority medication interventions based on emerging data collected in real time. Check this screen throughout your period of care to avoid missing critical information related to recently ordered or STAT medications.

- Clicking on **Patient Care** opens up three specific learning environments within the patient room: **Physical Assessment**, **Nurse-Client Interactions**, and **Medication Administration**.

- To perform a **Physical Assessment**, choose a body area (such as **Head & Neck**) from the column of yellow buttons. This activates a list of system subcategories for that body area (e.g., see **Sensory**, **Neurologic**, etc. in the green boxes). After you select the system you wish to evaluate, a brief description of the assessment findings will appear in a box to the right. A still photo provides a "snapshot" of how an assessment of this area might be done or what the finding might look like. For every body area, you can also click on **Equipment** on the right side of the screen.

- To the right of the Physical Assessment icon is **Nurse-Client Interactions**. Clicking on this icon will reveal the times and titles of any videos available for viewing. (*Note:* If the video you wish to see is not listed, this means you have not yet reached the correct virtual time to view that video. Check the virtual clock; you may return to access the video once its designated time has occurred—as long as you do so within the same period of care. Or you can click on the fast-forward icon within the virtual clock to advance the time by 2-minute intervals. You will then need to click again on **Patient Care** and **Nurse-Client Interactions** to refresh the screen.) To view a listed video, click on the white arrow to the right of the video title. Use the control buttons below the video to start, stop, pause, rewind, or fast-forward the action or to mute the sound.

- **Medication Administration** is the pathway that allows you to review and administer medications to a patient after you have prepared them in the Medication Room. This process is also addressed further in the *How to Prepare Medications* section below and in *Medications* in the **Detailed Tour**. For additional hands-on practice, see *Reducing Medication Errors* below the **Quick Tour** and **Detailed Tour** in your resources.

■ HOW TO CHANGE PATIENTS OR CHANGE PERIODS OF CARE

How to Change Patients or Periods of Care: To change patients, simply click on the new patient's room number. (You cannot receive a scorecard for a new patient, however, unless you have already selected that patient on the Patient List screen.) To change to a new period of care or to restart the virtual clock, click on **Leave the Floor** and then on **Restart the Program**.

Floor Menu

[hand/Eval icon]	**Look at your Preceptor's Evaluation.** Evaluations provide feedback on the work you completed during patient care. If you choose the Preceptor's Evaluation you will no longer be able to return to the floor.
[mug/door icon]	**Take a break.** Time will be stopped until you wish to return to the simulation.
[arrow icon]	**Restart the program.** If you restart, all data from your work in the current Period of Care will be erased.
CREDITS	**View Credits.** Take a look at the list of professionals who took part in the creation of this software suite.

0737   Return to Nurses' Station

■ HOW TO PREPARE MEDICATIONS

From the Nurses' Station or the patient's room, you can access the Medication Room by clicking on the icon in the tool bar at the bottom of your screen to the left of the patient room numbers.

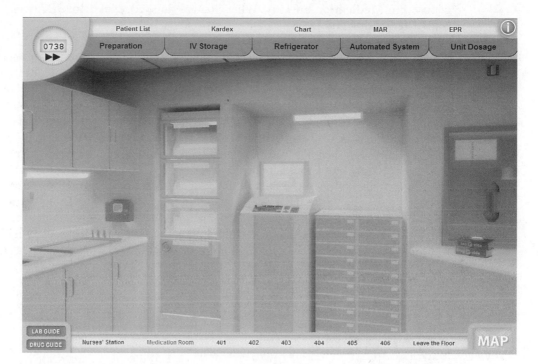

In the Medication Room you have access to the following (from left to right):

- A preparation area is located on the counter under the cabinets. To begin the medication preparation process, click on the tray on the counter or click on the **Preparation** icon at the top of the screen. The next screen leads you through a specific sequence (called the Preparation Wizard) to prepare medications one at a time for administration to a patient. However, no medication has been selected at this time. We will do this while working with a patient in *A Detailed Tour*. To exit this screen, click on **View Medication Room**.

- To the right of the cabinets (and above the refrigerator), IV storage bins are provided. Click on the bins themselves or on the **IV Storage** icon at the top of the screen. The bins are labeled **Microinfusion**, **Small Volume**, and **Large Volume**. Click on an individual bin to see a list of its contents. If you needed to prepare an IV medication at this time, you could click on the medication and its label would appear to the right under the patient's name. (*Note:* You can **Open** and **Close** any medication label by clicking the appropriate icon.) Next, you would click **Put Medication on Tray**. If you ever change your mind or decide that you have put the incorrect medication on the tray, you can reverse your actions by highlighting the medication on the tray and then clicking **Put Medication in Bin**. Click **Close Bin** in the right bottom corner to exit. **View Medication Room** brings you back to a full view of the entire room.

- A refrigerator is located under the IV storage bins to hold any medications that must be stored below room temperature. Click on the refrigerator door or on the **Refrigerator** icon at the top of the screen. Then click on the close-up view of the door to access the medications. When you are finished, click **Close Door** and then **View Medication Room**.

- To prepare controlled substances, click the **Automated System** icon at the top of the screen or click the computer monitor located to the right of the IV storage bins. A login screen will appear; your name and password are automatically filled in. Click **Login**. Select the patient for whom you wish to access medications; then select the correct medication drawer to open (they are stored alphabetically). Click **Open Drawer**, highlight the proper medication, and choose **Put Medication on Tray**. When you are finished, click **Close Drawer** and then **View Medication Room**.

- Next to the Automated System is a set of drawers identified by patient room number. To access these, click on the drawers or on the **Unit Dosage** icon at the top of the screen. This provides a close-up view of the drawers. To open a drawer, click on the room number of the patient you are working with. Next, click on the medication you would like to prepare for the patient, and a label will appear, listing the medication strength, units, and dosage per unit. To exit, click **Close Drawer**; then click **View Medication Room**.

At any time, you can learn about a medication you wish to prepare for a patient by clicking on the **Drug** icon in the bottom left corner of the medication room screen or by clicking the **Drug Guide** book on the counter to the right of the unit dosage drawers. The **Drug Guide** provides information about the medications commonly included in nursing drug handbooks. Nutritional supplements and maintenance intravenous fluid preparations are not included. Highlight a medication in the alphabetical list; relevant information about the drug will appear in the screen below. To exit, click **Return to Medication Room**.

To access the MAR from the Medication Room and to review the medications ordered for a patient, click on the **MAR** icon located in the tool bar at the top of your screen and then click on the correct tab for your patient's room number. You may also click the **Review MAR** icon in the tool bar at the bottom of your screen from inside each medication storage area.

After you have chosen and prepared medications, go to the patient's room to administer them by clicking on the room number in the bottom tool bar. Inside the patient's room, click **Patient Care** and then **Medication Administration** and follow the proper administration sequence.

■ PRECEPTOR'S EVALUATIONS

When you have finished a session, click on **Leave the Floor** to go to the Floor Menu. At this point, you can click on the top icon (**Look at Your Preceptor's Evaluation**) to receive a scorecard that provides feedback on the work you completed during patient care.

Floor Menu

Look at your Preceptor's Evaluation.
Evaluations provide feedback on the work you completed during patient care. If you choose the Preceptor's Evaluation you will no longer be able to return to the floor.

Take a break.
Time will be stopped until you wish to return to the simulation.

Restart the program.
If you restart, all data from your work in the current Period of Care will be erased.

View Credits.
Take a look at the list of professionals who took part in the creation of this software suite.

0737

Return to Nurses' Station

Evaluations are available for each patient you selected when you signed in for the current period of care. Click on the **Medication Scorecard** icon to see an example.

Medication Scorecard

Name:	Selma Brion	Evaluation For: Piya Jordan, Period of Care 1
Start Time:	0730	
End Time:	0731	

Instructions

Table A shows the medications that should have been administered to **Piya Jordan** and also shows if you gave those medications as ordered during this period of care. Table B lists the medications that you administered incorrectly: **Wrong Dosage, Wrong Route/Method/Site, or Wrong Time**. Compare Tables A and B to see where you made errors. Table C lists how often you accessed patient's medical records, as well as listing the times that you checked critical patient information, such as; Arm Band, Allergy Band, Clinical Update, and Vital Signs. Table D lists all other medications administered to other patients during this period of care. Use the information in Table D to determine if you administered a medication to the wrong patient.

Table A: Medications that should have been administered to **Piya Jordan** during this period of care.

Medication	Total Dosage	Route/Method/Site	Time	√ / X
Digoxin	0.5 mL	IV / Direct injection (push) / Peripheral IV	0730-0815	√
Morphine sulfate	30 mL	IV / Patient controlled analgesia / Peripheral IV	0730-0815	X
Potassium chloride	20 mEq in 250 mL NS	IV / Intermittent infusion / Peripheral IV	0730-0815	X

√ = Correct　X = Incorrect

Print		Return to Evaluations

The scorecard compares the medications you administered to a patient during a period of care with what should have been administered. Table A lists the correct medications. Table B lists any medications that were administered incorrectly.

Remember, not every medication listed on the MAR should necessarily be given. For example, a patient might have an allergy to a drug that was ordered, or a medication might have been improperly transcribed to the MAR. Predetermined medication "errors" embedded within the program challenge you to exercise critical thinking skills and professional judgment when deciding to administer a medication, just as you would in a real hospital. Use all your available resources, such as the patient's chart and the MAR, to make your decision.

Table C lists the resources that were available to assist you in medication administration. It also documents whether and when you accessed these resources. For example, did you check the patient armband or perform a check of vital signs? If so, when?

You can click **Print** to get a copy of this report if needed. When you have finished reviewing the scorecard, click **Return to Evaluations** and then **Return to Menu**.

■ FLOOR MAP

To get a general sense of your location within the hospital, you can click on the **Map** icon found in the lower right corner of most of the screens in the *Virtual Clinical Excursions—Medical-Surgical* program. (*Note:* If you are following this quick tour step by step, you will need to **Restart the Program** from the Floor Menu, sign in again, and go to the Nurses' Station to access the map.) When you click the **Map** icon, a floor map appears, showing the layout of the floor you are currently on, as well as a directory of the patients and services on that floor. As you move your cursor over the directory list, the location of each room is highlighted on the map (and vice versa). The floor map can be accessed from the Nurses' Station, Medication Room, and each patient's room.

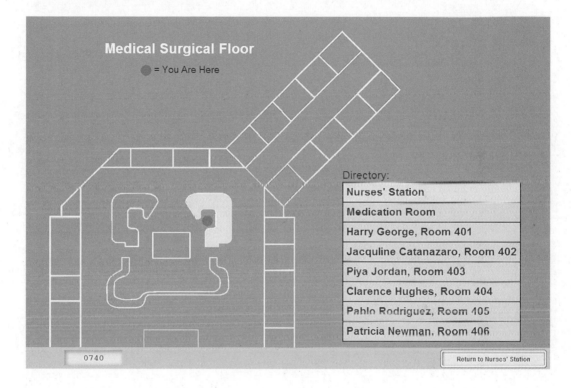

A DETAILED TOUR

If you wish to more thoroughly understand the capabilities of *Virtual Clinical Excursions—Medical-Surgical*, take a detailed tour by completing the following section. During this tour, we will work with a specific patient to introduce you to all the different components and learning opportunities available within the software.

■ WORKING WITH A PATIENT

Sign in for Period of Care 1 (0730-0815). From the Patient List, select Piya Jordan and Pablo Rodriguez; however, do not go to the Nurses' Station yet.

Patient List

	Patient Name	Room	MRN	Clinical Report
☐	Harry George	401	1868054	Get Report
☐	Jacquline Catanazaro	402	1868048	Get Report
☑	Piya Jordan	403	1868092	Get Report
☐	Clarence Hughes	404	1868011	Get Report
☑	Pablo Rodriguez	405	1868088	Get Report
☐	Patricia Newman	406	1868097	Get Report

Please select all the patients you will be caring for this period of care. Once you have exited the patient list, you will not be able to change your current selections or select new patients to care for.

0730   Go to Nurses' Station

■ REPORT

In hospitals, when one shift ends and another begins, the outgoing nurse who attended a patient will give a verbal and sometimes a written summary of that patient's condition to the incoming nurse who will assume care for the patient. This summary is called a report and is an important source of data to provide an overview of a patient. Your first task is to get the clinical report on Piya Jordan. To do this, click **Get Report** in the far right column in this patient's row. From a brief review of this summary, identify the problems and areas of concern that you will need to address for this patient.

When you have finished noting any areas of concern, click **Go to Nurses' Station**.

■ CHARTS

You can access Piya Jordan's chart from the Nurses' Station or from the patient's room (403). From the Nurses' Station, click on the chart rack or on the **Chart** icon in the tool bar at the top of your screen. Next, click on the chart labeled **403** to open the medical record for Piya Jordan. Click on the **Emergency Department** tab to view a record of why this patient was admitted.

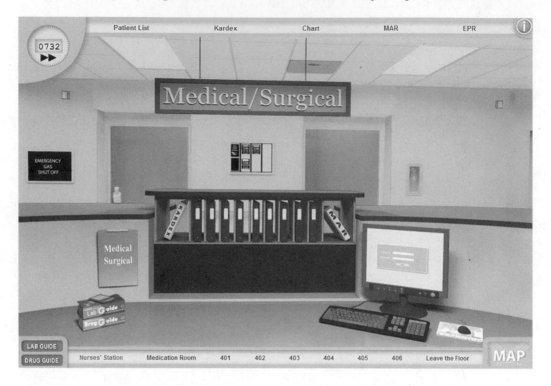

How many days has Piya Jordan been in the hospital?

What tests were done upon her arrival in the Emergency Department and why?

What was her reason for admission?

You should also click on **Diagnostic Reports** to learn what additional tests or procedures were performed and when. Finally, review the **Nursing Admission** and **History and Physical** to learn about the health history of this patient. When you are done reviewing the chart, click **Return to Nurses' Station**.

■ MEDICATIONS

Open the Medication Administration Record (MAR) by clicking on the **MAR** icon in the tool bar at the top of your screen. *Remember:* The MAR automatically opens to the first occupied room number on the floor—which is not necessarily your patient's room number! Since you need to access Piya Jordan's MAR, click on tab **403** (her room number). Always make sure you are giving the *Right Drug to the Right Patient!*

Examine the list of medications ordered for Piya Jordan. In the table below, list the medications that need to be given during this period of care (0730-0815). For each medication, note the dosage, route, and time to be given.

Time	Medication	Dosage	Route

Click on **Return to Nurses' Station**. Next, click on **403** on the bottom tool bar and then verify that you are indeed in Piya Jordan's room. Select **Clinical Alerts** (the icon to the right of Initial Observations) to check for any emerging data that might affect your medication administration priorities. Next, go to the patient's chart (click on the **Chart** icon; then click on **403**). When the chart opens, select the **Physician's Orders** tab.

Review the orders. Have any new medications been ordered? Return to the MAR (click **Return to Room 403**; then click **MAR**). Verify that any new medications have been correctly transcribed to the MAR. Mistakes are sometimes made in the transcription process in the hospital setting, and it is sound practice to double-check any new order.

Are there any patient assessments you will need to perform before administering these medications? If so, return to Room 403 and click on **Patient Care** and then **Physical Assessment** to complete those assessments before proceeding.

Now click on the **Medication Room** icon in the tool bar at the bottom of your screen to locate and prepare the medications for Piya Jordan.

In the Medication Room, you must access the medications for Piya Jordan from the specific dispensing system in which each medication is stored. Locate each medication that needs to be given in this time period and click on **Put Medication on Tray** as appropriate. (*Hint:* Look in **Unit Dosage** drawer first.) When you are finished, click on **Close Drawer** and then on **View Medication Room**. Now click on the medication tray on the counter on the left side of the medication room screen to begin preparing the medications you have selected. (*Remember:* You can also click **Preparation** in the tool bar at the top of the screen.)

In the preparation area, you should see a list of the medications you put on the tray in the previous steps. Click on the first medication and then click **Prepare**. Follow the onscreen instructions of the Preparation Wizard, providing any data requested. As an example, let's follow the preparation process for digoxin, one of the medications due to be administered to Piya Jordan during this period of care. To begin, click to select **Digoxin**; then click **Prepare**. Now work through the Preparation Wizard sequence as detailed below:

> Amount of medication in the ampule: 2 mL.
> Enter the amount of medication you will draw up into a syringe: **0.5** mL.
> Click **Next**.
> Select the patient you wish to set aside the medication for: **Room 403, Piya Jordan**.
> Click **Finish**.
> Click **Return to Medication Room**.

Preparation Wizard

Select the patient you wish to set aside the medication for:

Room 401, Harry George

Room 402, Jacquline Catanazaro

Room 403, Piya Jordan

Room 404, Clarence Hughes

Room 405, Pablo Rodriguez

Confirm that the information contained on the medication label (to the right) is correct and press "Finish" to prepare the medication.

Any leftover medication will be moved to the "leftover" list in your medication lists and can be disposed of or put back into medication systems from there.

Previous   Finish

CLOSE

Medication set aside for:
Room 403, Piya Jordan

Digoxin

Strength: 0.25 mg/mL

Units: 1 syringe

Dosage/Unit: 0.5 mL/syringe

LAB GUIDE
DRUG GUIDE   0733   Review MAR   Review Your Medications   View Medication Room

Follow this same basic process for the other medications due to be administered to Piya Jordan during this period of care. (*Hint:* Look in **IV Storage** and **Automated System**.)

PREPARATION WIZARD EXCEPTIONS

- Some medications in *Virtual Clinical Excursions—Medical-Surgical* are preprepared by the pharmacy (e.g., IV antibiotics) and taken to the patient room as a whole. This is common practice in most hospitals.
- Blood products are not administered by students through the *Virtual Clinical Excursions—Medical-Surgical* simulations since blood administration follows specific protocols not covered in this program.
- The *Virtual Clinical Excursions—Medical-Surgical* simulations do not allow for mixing more than one type of medication, such as regular and Lente insulins, in the same syringe. In the clinical setting, when multiple types of insulin are ordered for a patient, the regular insulin is drawn up first, followed by the longer-acting insulin. Insulin is always administered in a special unit-marked syringe.

Now return to Room 403 (click on **403** on the bottom tool bar) to administer Piya Jordan's medications.

At any time during the medication administration process, you can perform a further review of systems, take vital signs, check information contained within the chart, or verify patient identity and allergies. Inside Piya Jordan's room, click **Take Vital Signs**. (*Note:* These findings change over time to reflect the temporal changes you would find in a patient similar to Piya Jordan.)

When you have gathered all the data you need, click on **Patient Care** and then select **Medication Administration**. Any medications you prepared in the previous steps should be listed on the left side of your screen. Let's continue the administration process with the digoxin ordered for Piya Jordan. Click to highlight **Digoxin** in the list of medications. Next, click on the down arrow to the right of **Select** and choose **Administer** from the drop-down menu. This will activate the Administration Wizard. Complete the Wizard sequence as follows:

- Route: **IV**
- Method: **Direct Injection**
- Site: **Peripheral IV**
- Click **Administer to Patient** arrow.
- Would you like to document this administration in the MAR? **Yes**
- Click **Finish** arrow.

Your selections are recorded by a tracking system and evaluated on a Medication Scorecard stored under Preceptor's Evaluations. This scorecard can be viewed, printed, and given to your instructor. To access the Preceptor's Evaluations, click on **Leave the Floor**. When the Floor Menu appears, select **Look at Your Preceptor's Evaluation**. Then click on **Medication Scorecard** inside the box with Piya Jordan's name (see example on the following page).

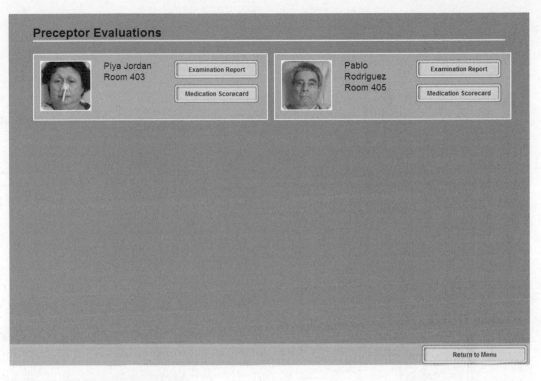

■ MEDICATION SCORECARD

- First, review Table A. Was digoxin given correctly? Did you give the other medications as ordered?
- Table B shows you which (if any) medications you gave incorrectly.
- Table C addresses the resources used for Piya Jordan. Did you access the patient's chart, MAR, EPR, or Kardex as needed to make safe medication administration decisions?
- Did you check the patient's armband to verify her identity? Did you check whether your patient had any known allergies to medications? Were vital signs taken?

When you have finished reviewing the scorecard, click **Return to Evaluations** and then **Return to Menu**.

■ **VITAL SIGNS**

Vital signs, often considered the traditional "signs of life," include body temperature, heart rate, respiratory rate, blood pressure, oxygen saturation of the blood, and pain level.

Inside Piya Jordan's room, click **Take Vital Signs**. (*Note:* If you are following this detailed tour step by step, you will need to **Restart the Program** from the Floor Menu, sign in again for Period of Care 1, and navigate to Room 403.) Collect vital signs for this patient and record them below. Note the time at which you collected each of these data. (*Remember:* You can take vital signs at any time. The data change over time to reflect the temporal changes you would find in a patient similar to Piya Jordan.)

Vital Signs	Findings/Time
Blood pressure	
O$_2$ saturation	
Temperature	
Heart rate	
Respiratory rate	
Pain rating	

After you are done, click on the **EPR** icon located in the tool bar at the top of the screen. Your username and password are automatically provided. Click on **Login** to enter the EPR. To access Piya Jordan's records, click on the down arrow next to Patient and choose her room number, **403**. Select **Vital Signs** as the category. Next, in the empty time column on the far right, record the vital signs data you just collected in Piya Jordan's room. If you need help with this process, refer to the Electronic Patient Record (EPR) section of the Quick Tour. Now compare these findings with the data you collected earlier for this patient's vital signs. Use these earlier findings to establish a baseline for each of the vital signs.

    a.   Are any of the data you collected significantly different from the baseline for a particular vital sign?

       Circle One: Yes   No

    b.   If "Yes," which data are different?

■ PHYSICAL ASSESSMENT

After you have finished examining the EPR for vital signs, click **Exit EPR** to return to Room 403. Click **Patient Care** and then **Physical Assessment**. Think about the information you received in the report at the beginning of this shift, as well as what you may have learned about this patient from the chart. Based on this, what area(s) of examination should you pay most attention to at this time? Is there any equipment you should be monitoring? Conduct a physical assessment of the body areas and systems that you consider priorities for Piya Jordan. For example, select **Head & Neck**; then click on and assess **Sensory** and **Lymphatic**. Complete any other assessment(s) you think are necessary at this time. In the following table, record the data you collected during this examination.

Area of Examination	Findings
Head & Neck Sensory	
Head & Neck Lymphatic	

After you have finished collecting these data, return to the EPR. Compare the data that were already in the record with those you just collected.

a.   Are any of the data you collected significantly different from the baselines for this patient?

Circle One: Yes   No

b.   If "Yes," which data are different?

■ **NURSE-CLIENT INTERACTIONS**

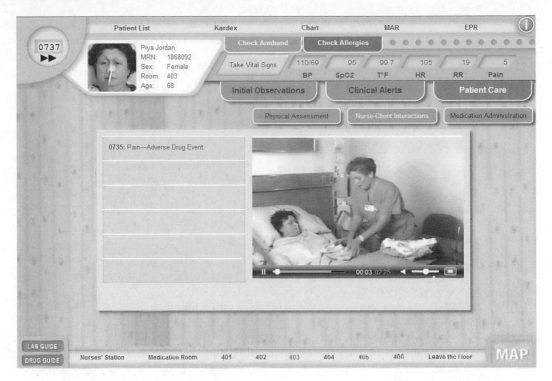

Click on **Patient Care** from inside Piya Jordan's room (403). Now click on **Nurse-Client Interactions** to access a short video titled **Pain—Adverse Drug Event**, which is available for viewing at or after 0735 (based on the virtual clock in the upper left corner of your screen; see *Note* below). To begin the video, click on the white arrow next to its title. You will observe a nurse communicating with Piya Jordan and her daughter. There are many variations of nursing practice, some exemplifying "best" practice and some not. Note whether the nurse in this interaction displays professional behavior and compassionate care. Are her words congruent with what is going on with the patient? Does this interaction "feel right" to you? If not, how would you handle this situation differently? Explain.

Note: If the video you wish to view is not listed, this means you have not yet reached the correct virtual time to view that video. Check the virtual clock; you may return to access the video once its designated time has occurred—as long as you do so within the same period of care. Or you can click on the fast-forward icon within the virtual clock to advance the time by 2-minute intervals. You will then need to click again on **Patient Care** and **Nurse-Client Interactions** to refresh the screen.

At least one Nurse-Client Interactions video is available during each period of care. Viewing these videos can help you learn more about what is occurring with a patient at a certain time and also prompt you to discern between nurse communications that are ideal and those that need improvement. Compassionate care and the ability to communicate clearly are essential components of delivering quality nursing care, and it is during your clinical time that you will begin to refine these skills.

■ COLLECTING AND EVALUATING DATA

Each of the activities you perform in the Patient Care environment generates a significant amount of assessment data. Remember that after you collect data, you can record your findings in the EPR. You can also review the EPR, patient's chart, videos, and MAR at any time. You will get plenty of practice collecting and then evaluating data in context of the patient's course.

Now, here's an important question for you:

> Did the previous sequence of exercises provide the most efficient way to assess Piya Jordan?

For example, you went to the patient's room to get vital signs, then back to the EPR to enter data and compare your findings with extant data. Next, you went back to the patient's room to do a physical examination, then again back to the EPR to enter and review data. If this back-and-forth process of data collection and recording seemed inefficient, remember the following:

- Plan all of your nursing activities to maximize efficiency, while at the same time optimizing the quality of patient care. (Think about what data you might need before performing certain tasks. For example, do you need to check a heart rate before administering a cardiac medication or check an IV site before starting an infusion?)

- You collect a tremendous amount of data when you work with a patient. Very few people can accurately remember all these data for more than a few minutes. Develop efficient assessment skills, and record data as soon as possible after collecting them.

- Assessment data are only the starting point for the nursing process.

Make a clear distinction between these first exercises and how you actually provide nursing care. These initial exercises were designed to involve you actively in the use of different software components. This workbook focuses on sensible practices for implementing the nursing process in ways that ensure the highest-quality care of patients.

Most important, remember that a human being changes through time, and that these changes include both the physical and psychosocial facets of a person as a living organism. Think about this for a moment. Some patients may change physically in a very short time (a patient with emerging myocardial infarction) or more slowly (a patient with a chronic illness). Patients' overall physical and psychosocial conditions may improve or deteriorate. They may have effective coping skills and familial support, or they may feel alone and full of despair. In fact, each individual is a complex mix of physical and psychosocial elements, and at least some of these elements usually change through time.

Thus it is crucial that you *DO NOT* think of the nursing process as a simple one-time, five-step procedure consisting of assessment, nursing diagnosis, planning, implementation, and evaluation. Rather, the nursing process should be utilized as a creative and systematic approach to delivering nursing care. Furthermore, because all living organisms are constantly changing, we must apply the nursing process over and over. Each time we follow the nursing process for an individual patient, we refine our understanding of that patient's physical and psychosocial conditions based on collection and analysis of many different types of data. *Virtual Clinical Excursions—Medical-Surgical* will help you develop both the creativity and the systematic approach needed to become a nurse who is equipped to deliver the highest-quality care to all patients.

REDUCING MEDICATION ERRORS

Earlier in the detailed tour, you learned the basic steps of medication preparation and administration. The following simulations will allow you to practice those skills further—with an increased emphasis on reducing medication errors by using the Medication Scorecard to evaluate your work.

Sign in to work at Pacific View Regional Hospital for Period of Care 1. (*Note:* If you are already working with another patient or during another period of care, click on **Leave the Floor** and then **Restart the Program**; then sign in.)

From the Patient List, select Clarence Hughes. Then click on **Go to Nurses' Station**. Complete the following steps to prepare and administer medications to Clarence Hughes.

- Click on **Medication Room** on the tool bar at the bottom of your screen.
- Click on **MAR** and then on tab **404** to determine medications that have been ordered for Clarence Hughes. (*Note:* You may click on **Review MAR** at any time to verify the correct medication order. Always remember to check the patient name on the MAR to make sure you have the correct patient's record. You must click on the correct room number tab within the MAR.) Click on **Return to Medication Room** after reviewing the correct MAR.
- Click on **Unit Dosage** (or on the Unit Dosage cabinet); from the close-up view, click on drawer **404**.
- Select the medications you would like to administer. After each selection, click **Put Medication on Tray**. When you are finished selecting medications, click **Close Drawer** and then **View Medication Room**.
- Click on **Automated System** (or on the Automated System unit itself). Click **Login**.
- On the next screen, specify the correct patient and drawer location.
- Select the medication you would like to administer and click on **Put Medication on Tray**. Repeat this process if you wish to administer other medications from the Automated System.
- When you are finished, click **Close Drawer** and **View Medication Room**.
- From the Medication Room, click on **Preparation** (or on the preparation tray).
- From the list of medications on your tray, highlight the correct medication to administer and click **Prepare**.
- This activates the Preparation Wizard. Supply any requested information; then click **Next**.
- Now select the correct patient to receive this medication and click **Finish**.
- Repeat the previous three steps until all medications that you want to administer are prepared.
- You can click on **Review Your Medications** and then on **Return to Medication Room** when ready. Once you are back in the Medication Room, go directly to Clarence Hughes' room by clicking on **404** at bottom of screen.
- Inside the patient's room, administer the medication, utilizing the six rights of medication administration. After you have collected the appropriate assessment data and are ready for administration, click **Patient Care** and then **Medication Administration**. Verify that the correct patient and medication(s) appear in the left-hand window. Highlight the first medication you wish to administer; then click the down arrow next to Select. From the drop-down menu, select **Administer** and complete the Administration Wizard by providing any information requested. When the Wizard stops asking for information, click **Administer to Patient**. Specify **Yes** when asked whether this administration should be recorded in the MAR. Finally, click **Finish**.

■ **SELF-EVALUATION**

Now let's see how you did during your medication administration!

• Click on **Leave the Floor** at the bottom of your screen. From the Floor Menu, select **Look at Your Preceptor's Evaluation**. Then click **Medication Scorecard**.

The following exercises will help you identify medication errors, investigate possible reasons for these errors, and reduce or prevent medication errors in the future.

1. Start by examining Table A. These are the medications you should have given to Clarence Hughes during this period of care. If each of the medications in Table A has a ✓ by it, then you made no errors. Congratulations!

If any medication has an X by it, then you made one or more medication errors.

Compare Tables A and B to determine which of the following types of errors you made: Wrong Dose, Wrong Route/Method/Site, or Wrong Time. Follow these steps:
   a. Find medications in Table A that were given incorrectly.
   b. Now see if those same medications are in Table B, which shows what you actually administered to Clarence Hughes.
   c. Comparing Tables A and B, match the Strength, Dose, Route/Method/Site, and Time for each medication you administered incorrectly.
   d. Then, using the form below, list the medications given incorrectly and mark the errors you made for each medication.

Medication	Strength	Dosage	Route	Method	Site	Time
	❑	❑	❑	❑	❑	❑
	❑	❑	❑	❑	❑	❑
	❑	❑	❑	❑	❑	❑
	❑	❑	❑	❑	❑	❑

2. To help you reduce future medication errors, consider the following list of possible reasons for errors.

   • Did not check drug against MAR for correct medication, correct dose, correct patient, correct route, correct time, correct documentation.
   • Did not check drug dose against MAR three times.
   • Did not open the unit dose package in the patient's room.
   • Did not correctly identify the patient using two identifiers.
   • Did not administer the drug on time.
   • Did not verify patient allergies.
   • Did not check the patient's current condition or vital sign parameters.
   • Did not consider why the patient would be receiving this drug.
   • Did not question why the drug was in the patient's drawer.
   • Did not check the physician's order and/or check with the pharmacist when there was a question about the drug or dose.
   • Did not verify that no adverse effects had occurred from a previous dose.

Based on the list of possibilities you just reviewed, determine how you made each error and record the reason in the form below:

Medication	Reason for Error

3. Look again at Table B. Are there medications listed that are not in Table A? If so, you gave a medication to Clarence Hughes that he should not have received. Complete the following exercises to help you understand how such an error might have been made.

   a. Perhaps you gave a medication that was on Clarence Hughes' MAR for this period of care, without recognizing that a change had occurred in the patient's condition, which should have caused you to reconsider. Review patient records as necessary and complete the following form:

Medication	Possible Reasons Not to Give This Medication

   b. Another possibility is that you gave Clarence Hughes a medication that should have been given at a different time. Check his MAR and complete the form below to determine whether you made a Wrong Time error:

Medication	Given to Clarence Hughes at What Time	Should Have Been Given at What Time

c. Maybe you gave another patient's medication to Clarence Hughes. In this case, you made a Wrong Patient error. Check the MARs of other patients and use the form below to determine whether you made this type of error:

Medication	Given to Clarence Hughes	Should Have Been Given to

4. The Medication Scorecard provides some other interesting sources of information. For example, if there is a medication selected for Clarence Hughes but it was not given to him, there will be an X by that medication in Table A, but it will not appear in Table B. In that case, you might have given this medication to some other patient, which is another type of Wrong Patient error. To investigate further, look at Table D, which lists the medications you gave to other patients. See whether you can find any medications ordered for Clarence Hughes that were given to another patient by mistake. However, before you make any decisions, be sure to cross-check the MAR for other patients because the same medication may have been ordered for multiple patients. Use the following form to record your findings:

Medication	Should Have Been Given to Clarence Hughes	Given by Mistake to

5. Now take some time to review the medication exercises you just completed. Use the form below to create an overall analysis of what you have learned. Once again, record each of the medication errors you made, including the type of each error. Then, for each error you made, indicate specifically what you would do differently to prevent this type of error from occurring again.

Medication	Type of Error	Error Prevention Tactic

Submit this form to your instructor if required as a graded assignment, or simply use these exercises to improve your understanding of medication errors and how to reduce them.

Name: _____   Date: _____

LESSON 1

Assessment of the Patient with Osteomyelitis

Reading Assignment: Care of the Patient with an Integumentary Disorder (Chapter 3)
Care of the Patient with a Musculoskeletal Disorder (Chapter 4)

Patient: Harry George, Room 401

Objectives:

1. Understand the basic functions of the musculoskeletal system.
2. Review the various types of arthritis.
3. Review risk factors for osteomyelitis.
4. Identify the clinical manifestations of osteomyelitis.
5. Discuss treatment options for the patient with osteomyelitis.

Exercise 1

Writing Activity

15 minutes

1. The skeletal system serves five major functions:

    a. The skeleton provides the body _____ that supports internal tissues and organs.

    b. The skeleton forms a _____ that protects many internal organs.

    c. Bones provide _____ for movement.

    d. The bones serve as storage areas for various _____.

    e. _____ (blood cell formation) takes place in the red bone marrow.

2. Match each type of body movement with its correct definition. (*Hint:* See Box 4-2 in your textbook.)

Type of Body Movement	Definition
_____ Abduction	a. Movement of the bone around its longitudinal axis
_____ Adduction	b. Movement that causes the bottom of the foot to be directed downward
_____ Dorsiflexion	
_____ Extension	c. Movement of certain joints that decreases the angle between two adjoining bones
_____ Flexion	d. Movement of the hand and forearm causing the palm to face downward or backward
_____ Plantar flexion	
_____ Pronation	e. Movement of an extremity toward the axis of the body
_____ Rotation	f. Movement of the hand and forearm that causes the palm to face upward or forward
_____ Supination	g. Movement of certain joints that increases the angle between two adjoining bones
	h. Movement of an extremity away from the midline of the body
	i. Movement that causes the top of the foot to elevate or tilt upward

3. Which muscles are responsible for movement of the lower extremities? Select all that apply.

   _____   Gluteus maximus

   _____   Soleus

   _____   Masseter

   _____   Orbicularis oris

   _____   Adductor longus

4. List the four most common types of arthritis.

5. The nurse conducts a teaching session for a patient diagnosed with gout. During the discussion, the nurse addresses dietary concerns. Which statements by the patient indicate the need for further instruction? Select all that apply.

   _____   "I should avoid hard liquor but can still indulge in beer or wine with my condition."

   _____   "Organ meats contain high levels of protein and will help in the management of my condition."

   _____   "I will need to avoid yeast-containing products."

   _____   "Certain seafood items may be problematic and will need to be avoided."

   _____   "I should limit my fluid intake during the flare-ups of my condition."

6. The nurse is reviewing the chart of a patient who is suspected of having rheumatoid arthritis. What findings would be consistent with the condition? Select all that apply.

   _____   Complete cell count that indicates a reduced white blood cell count

   _____   Bony knobs on the ends of the fingers

   _____   Familial history of rheumatoid arthritis

   _____   Patient complaints of tenderness of joints

   _____   Symmetrical involvement of joints

7. A female patient with a strong family history of osteoarthritis has voiced concerns about the disease. The patient asks what areas of the body are most often affected in her gender. What information can be provided by the nurse?
   a. Osteoarthritis affects the hips of women most often.
   b. Osteoarthritic changes are most often evident in the knees of women.
   c. Osteoarthritis affects the hands of women most often.
   d. Osteoarthritis is seen most often in the lumbosacral region of women most often.

8. Osteomyelitis is an infection of bone and/or bone marrow. What are the most common causes of osteomyelitis?

9. A variety of organisms may cause osteomyelitis. What is the most common causative agent?
   a. *Staphylococcus aureus*
   b. *Streptococcus viridans*
   c. *Escherichia coli*
   d. *Neisseria gonorrhoeae*

10. How is osteomyelitis treated?

Exercise 2

Virtual Hospital Activity

45 minutes

- Sign in to work at Pacific View Regional Hospital for Period of Care 1. (*Note:* If you are already in the virtual hospital from a previous exercise, click **Leave the Floor** and then **Restart the Program** to get to the sign-in window.)
- From the Patient List, select Harry George (Room 401).
- Click **Get Report** and read the Clinical Report.
- Click **Go to Nurses' Station**; then click **401** to enter Harry George's room.
- Click **Patient Care** and complete a head-to-toe assessment.

1. When you are assessing Harry George's affected extremity, which factors should you include in the assessment?

2. Harry George was admitted with a diagnosis of osteomyelitis. What findings support this diagnosis?

3. How does the affected extremity appear?

4. How does the assessment of the left (affected) leg differ from that of the right?

5. What other clinical manifestations may accompany a diagnosis of osteomyelitis?

6. How should the affected extremity be positioned?

7. During the head-to-toe assessment, Harry George asks the nurse how long it will take before he "no longer has this nasty infection in his bones." What response by the nurse is most appropriate?
   a. "Once you complete this course of antibiotic therapy, you should have this infection beat."
   b. "You may have this infection for at least another year."
   c. "An infection of the bone is difficult to treat and may be a factor for your entire life."
   d. "It takes at least 6 months to know if and when you will be free of infection."

- Click **Take Vital Signs** and review the information provided.

8. Discuss any findings in Harry George's vital signs that may indicate the presence of infection.

- Click **Chart** at the top of the screen.
- Click **401** to view Harry George's chart.
- Click the **Consultations** tab.
- Review the report by the Wound Care Team.

9. Based on the description, what stage can best be used to classify Harry George's wound?
   a. Stage I
   b. Stage II
   c. Stage III
   d. Stage IV

10. What age-related changes will further affect Harry George's ability to achieve wound healing? Select all that apply.

   _____ Increases in tissue fluid

   _____ Reduced skin elasticity

   _____ Reductions in subcutaneous fat

   _____ Circulatory changes

11. Which diagnostic tests may be ordered to support a diagnosis of osteomyelitis? Select all that apply.

   _____ MRI

   _____ PET scan

   _____ Bone scan

   _____ X-rays

   _____ Serum electrolytes

   _____ Erythrocyte sedimentation rate

   _____ Blood cultures

   _____ Cultures of any drainage from open wounds

   _____ Complete blood count

- Still in Harry George's chart, click and review the **Laboratory Reports** and the **Diagnostic Reports** sections.

12. What diagnostic tests were ordered for Harry George to support the diagnosis of osteomyelitis?

13. Which lab results support the diagnosis?

14. What findings were reported in the x-ray and bone scan?

• Click the **History and Physical** tab and review this report.

15. Based on your review of Harry George's medical and social history, what risk factors for osteomyelitis does he have?

16. What will be assessed to determine the effectiveness of Harry George's treatment?

Let's jump ahead to a later period of care and check on Harry George's condition.

• Click **Return to Nurses' Station**.
• Click **Leave the Floor**.
• Click **Restart the Program**.
• Sign in to work at Pacific View Regional Hospital for Period of Care 3.
• Select Harry George from the Patient List.

- Click **Go to Nurses' Station**.
- Click **Chart**.
- Click **401**.
- Click the **Physician's Orders** tab and review the orders given.

17. What treatments have been ordered to manage Harry George's osteomyelitis?

18. What consultations have been ordered by the physician to assist in the management of Harry George's care?

- Click **Consultations**.
- Review the Wound Care Team report.

19. What concerns did the Wound Care Team reveal that are seen as detriments to the healing of Harry George's wound? How can these concerns present problems?

20. The nurse is planning to assist Harry George in the selection of foods that are rich in elements to promote wound healing. Which vitamins should the nurse recognize as vital to his healing? Select all that apply.

_____ Vitamin A

_____ Vitamin B

_____ Vitamin C

_____ Vitamin D

_____ Calcium

_____ Iron

_____ Magnesium

21. What interventions can the nurse implement to manage the concerns of the Wound Care Team?

- Click **Return to Nurses' Station**.
- Click **MAR** and then click tab **401**.
- Review the information given.

22. These medications have been prescribed by Harry George's physician. Which are intended to manage his osteomyelitis? Select all that apply.

_____   Gentamicin 20 mg IV

_____   Thiamine 100 mg PO/IM

_____   Glyburide 1.25 mg PO

_____   Cefotaxime 2 g IV

_____   Phenytoin sodium 100 mg

2

Care of the Patient Experiencing Comorbid Conditions (Musculoskeletal and Endocrine)

Reading Assignment: Care of the Patient with an Endocrine Disorder (Chapter 11)

Patient: Harry George, Room 401

Objectives:

1. Describe the functions of the endocrine system.
2. Describe the use of a sliding insulin scale.
3. Explain how type 1 and type 2 diabetes are similar and how they differ.
4. List disorders of the endocrine system.
5. Describe the tests used to assess for the presence of diabetes.

Exercise 1

Writing Activity

30 minutes

1. Which statements are true regarding the role and/or function of the endocrine and exocrine systems? Select all that apply.

   _____ Endocrine glands are ductless glands.

   _____ Exocrine glands are responsible for reproductive functioning.

   _____ Endocrine glands release their secretions directly into the bloodstream.

   _____ The endocrine system secretes hormones.

   _____ Exocrine glands assist with maintaining homeostasis for the body.

2. The _____ is considered the "master gland" of the endocrine system.

3. _____ is the means by which the endocrine system maintains homeostasis.

4. Match each disorder of the pituitary gland with its correct description.

Disorder of the Pituitary Gland	Description
_____ Acromegaly	a. A transient or permanent metabolic disorder of the posterior pituitary in which ADH is deficient
_____ Gigantism	
_____ Dwarfism	b. A disorder in which the pituitary gland releases too much ADH and, in response, the kidneys reabsorb more water
_____ Diabetes insipidus	c. An overproduction of somatotropin in the adult
_____ Syndrome of inappropriate secretion of antidiuretic hormone (SIADH)	d. A condition in which there is a deficiency in growth hormone
	e. A condition that usually results from an oversecretion of growth hormone

5. What is diabetes?

6. For each characteristic listed below, identify whether it is a characteristic of (a) type 1 diabetes mellitus, (b) type 2 diabetes mellitus, or (c) both type 1 and type 2 diabetes mellitus.

Characteristic	Type of Diabetes
_____ Usually associated with individuals under age 30	a. Type 1 diabetes mellitus
_____ Underweight	b. Type 2 diabetes mellitus
_____ Overweight	c. Both type 1 and type 2 diabetes mellitus
_____ May be controlled with oral agents	
_____ Incidence of complications	
_____ Gradual onset	

7. A patient recently diagnosed with diabetes mellitus asks the nurse about potential causes. The nurse correctly recognizes that which factors may be considered to have a causative relationship with the disease? Select all that apply.

_____ Obesity

_____ Autoimmune disorder development

_____ Ethnicity

_____ Lifestyle

_____ Caucasian

_____ Genetic factors

8. Match each diagnostic test for diabetes with its function. (*Hint:* See Box 11-2 in your textbook.)

Diagnostic Test	Function
_____ Fasting blood glucose	a. Test used to determine the presence of either type 1 or type 2 diabetes mellitus
_____ Postprandial blood glucose	b. The administration of a carbohydrate solution followed by drawing a blood specimen to assess the level of blood glucose hours later
_____ Glycosylated hemoglobin	c. Drawing of a blood sample after a period of fasting, typically 8 hours
_____ C peptide	d. Used to measure the level of glucose that has been incorporated into the body's hemoglobin

9. Match each type of insulin with its correct onset of action after administration.

Type of Insulin	Onset of Action After Administration
_____ Humalog	a. 15-30 minutes
_____ Regular	b. 30-60 minutes
_____ NPH	c. 1-2 hours
_____ Lente (70/30)	d. 1-3 hours
_____ Lantus	e. 2-4 hours

10. Most available insulin is U/_____.

11. Indicate whether each statement is true or false.

   a. _____ Urine testing is the recommended way of monitoring glucose levels in the IDDM patient.

   b. _____ Lantus should never be mixed with regular insulin.

   c. _____ Patients with diabetes can choose between insulin or oral agents.

12. Insulin should be administered to the _____ tissue.

13. Which is the site with the fastest rate of insulin absorption?
   a. Abdomen
   b. Arms
   c. Thighs
   d. Buttocks

14. The loss of fat deposits as a result of insulin administration is known as

   _____.

15. The only insulin that can be administered intravenously is _____.

Exercise 2

Virtual Hospital Activity

30 minutes

- Sign in to work at Pacific View Regional Hospital for Period of Care 1. (*Note:* If you are already in the virtual hospital from a previous exercise, click **Leave the Floor** and then **Restart the Program** to get to the sign-in window.)
- From the Patient List, select Harry George (Room 401).
- Click **Get Report** and read the Clinical Report.
- Click **Go to Nurses' Station** and then click **Chart**.
- Click **401** to view Harry George's chart.
- Click the **Emergency Department** tab and review the information given.
- Click the **Laboratory Reports** tab and review the information given.

1. What was Harry George's plasma blood glucose upon his arrival at the emergency department?

2. Harry George's HbA1C is _____ .

3. Based on the HbA1C level, what inferences can be made about Harry George's typical blood glucose levels?
   a. Harry George's blood glucose levels are most often between 130 and 150 mg/dL.
   b. Harry George's blood glucose levels are most often between 150 and 175 mg/dL.
   c. Harry George's blood glucose levels are most often between 175 and 200 mg/dL.
   d. Harry George's blood glucose levels most often exceed 200 mg/dL.

4. What is the desired blood glucose level for a patient with diabetes?

5. Which type of diabetes does Harry George have?
   a. Diabetes insipidus
   b. Type 1 diabetes mellitus
   c. Type 2 diabetes mellitus
   d. Prediabetes

6. What medication does Harry George take at home to control his diabetes?

7. Which action best describes the mechanics of the drug you identified in the previous question?
   a. Stimulates the beta cells of the pancreas to release insulin
   b. Works to reduce hepatic glucose production
   c. Works to increase cell receptiveness to the body's natural insulin
   d. Inhibits glucose conversion to glucagon

8. In addition to his daily scheduled medications to control his diabetes, Harry George has a sliding scale. Describe the use of a sliding scale.

9. When caring for Harry George, the nurse notes that his blood glucose level is less than 150 mg/dL. What actions by the nurse are most appropriate? Select all that apply.

_____ Hold the prescribed dose of oral hypoglycemic medication.

_____ Provide him with a carbohydrate snack.

_____ Notify the health care provider.

_____ Document the findings.

_____ Administer the prescribed oral hypoglycemic medication.

10. During an illness what is the recommended frequency of blood glucose monitoring for the patient?
    a. Hourly
    b. Every 1 to 2 hours
    c. Every 4 hours
    d. Every 8 hours

11. What impact might illness have on Harry George's blood glucose?

12. How does Harry George's diabetes affect his health status? For which additional complications might he be at risk because of his diabetes?

- Click **Return to Nurses' Station**.
- Click **401** at the bottom of the screen to enter Harry George's room.
- Click **Patient Care** and then **Nurse-Client Interactions**.
- Select and view the video titled **0735: Symptom Management**. (*Note:* Check the virtual clock to see whether enough time has elapsed. You can use the fast-forward feature to advance the time by 2-minute intervals if the video is not yet available. Then click again on **Patient Care** and **Nurse-Client Interactions** to refresh the screen.)

13. What nonverbal behaviors are displayed by the patient, indicating a problem that needs to be addressed?

14. During the talk between Harry George and his sitter, what needs and concerns are voiced?

- Click **Chart** and then **401** to view Harry George's chart.
- Click the **Physician's Orders** tab and review the orders.

15. What is the frequency of Harry George's blood glucose assessments?

16. What type of dietary management is being implemented?

17. Which statement concerning Harry George's prescribed diet is correct?
    a. The diet will consist of three full meals per day to prevent snacking.
    b. The fat content should consist of no more than 30% of the caloric intake.
    c. 60% to 70 % of the calories in the diet should be from carbohydrates to ensure energy.
    d. Snacks should be avoided to reduce blood sugar fluctuations.

18. Harry George should be assessed for teaching needed in which areas?

- Click **Return to Room 401**.
- Click **Patient Care** and then **Nurse-Client Interactions**.
- Select and view the video titled **0755: Disease Management**. (*Note:* Check the virtual clock to see whether enough time has elapsed. You can use the fast-forward feature to advance the time by 2-minute intervals if the video is not yet available. Then click again on **Patient Care** and **Nurse-Client Interactions** to refresh the screen.)

19. While talking with his sitter, Harry George continues to voice the need for his own "medication." What technique does the sitter attempt to employ to manage this request?

LESSON 3

Developing a Plan of Care for the Patient with Osteomyelitis

Reading Assignment: Care of the Patient with a Musculoskeletal Disorder (Chapter 4)

Patient: Harry George, Room 401

Objectives:

1. Understand factors that affect pain management.
2. Identify nursing implications for the administration of narcotic analgesics.
3. Set priorities for the care of the patient with osteomyelitis.

Exercise 1

Virtual Hospital Activity

60 minutes

- Sign in to work at Pacific View Regional Hospital for Period of Care 2. (*Note:* If you are already in the virtual hospital from a previous exercise, click **Leave the Floor** and then **Restart the Program** to get to the sign-in window.)
- From the Patient List, select Harry George (Room 401).
- Click **Get Report** and read the Clinical Report.
- Click **Go to Nurses' Station** and then **401** to enter Harry George's room.
- Read the **Initial Observations**.
- Click **Patient Care** and complete a head-to-toe assessment.

1. What are the two primary priorities for Harry George's care at this time?

2. What elements of the assessment or the clinical report did you use to make this decision?

3. How has pain interfered with Harry George's recovery?

4. Is Harry George's pain a new problem or one that has been ongoing? Give a rationale for your response.

5. What nonpharmacologic interventions can be used to attempt to increase Harry George's level of comfort?

- Click **Patient Care** and then **Nurse-Client Interactions**.
- Select and view the video titled **1120: Wound Management**. (*Note:* Check the virtual clock to see whether enough time has elapsed. You can use the fast-forward feature to advance the time by 2-minute intervals if the video is not yet available. Then click again on **Patient Care** and **Nurse-Client Interactions** to refresh the screen.)

6. What behaviors demonstrated by Harry George further support his report of pain and his level of anxiety?

- Now select and view the video titled **1125: Injury Prevention**. (*Note:* Check the virtual clock to see whether enough time has elapsed. You can use the fast-forward feature to advance the time by 2-minute intervals if the video is not yet available. Then click again on **Patient Care** and **Nurse-Client Interactions** to refresh the screen.)

7. During the interaction with his sitter, Harry George continues to appear nervous. His movements reflect jitteriness, and his extremities are trembling. To what can these behaviors be attributed?

- Click **MAR** and then tab **401** to review Harry George's MAR.

8. The physician has prescribed chlordiazepoxide hydrochloride. Other than anxiety, what is an indication for the use of this medication?

9. Which nursing implications are indicated with the administration of chlordiazepoxide hydrochloride? Select all that apply.

   _____ Assess vital signs before administration.

   _____ Increase ambulation immediately after administration.

   _____ Administer cautiously in patients with liver impairments.

   _____ Institute safety precautions in regard to ambulation.

   _____ This medication may be used in patients who have recently ingested alcohol.

10. In addition to the chlordiazepoxide, what alternative(s) has the physician ordered to reduce Harry George's anxiety?

11. What factors will determine which of the medications should be given?

12. What medication has been ordered to manage Harry George's pain?

13. Does Harry George have any allergies that prevent him from being medicated with the drug prescribed? (*Hint:* Check his armband.)

14. Harry George's last dose of medication for pain was given at _____.

- Click **Return to Room 401**. Then click the **Drug** icon.
- Review the information provided for the medication you identified in question 12.

15. What elements of Harry George's medical/social history should be taken into consideration when administering this drug?

16. Are there any special administration precautions that must be observed when giving this medication IV push?

17. Are there any special considerations to address when administering this drug in conjunction with the other medications currently in use?

18. Identify any safety measures that should be observed after administration of this medication.

19. Is it time for Harry George to be medicated again for pain?

- Click **Return to Room 401**. Then click **Take Vital Signs**.

20. What are Harry George's vital signs? (*Note:* Exact findings will vary depending on the virtual time at which they are taken.)

    BP:

    SpO$_2$:

    T:

    HR:

    RR:

    Pain:

21. What impact has Harry George's pain had on his vital signs?

22. Are Harry George's vital signs within acceptable limits to administer the drug that has been ordered to manage his pain?

23. If Harry George is unable to take his prescribed medications, what action(s) would be appropriate?

LESSON 4

Postoperative Assessment

Reading Assignment: Care of the Surgical Patient (Chapter 2)
Care of the Patient with a Musculoskeletal Disorder (Chapter 4)

Patient: Clarence Hughes, Room 404

Objectives:

1. Define degenerative joint disease.
2. Identify the clinical signs and symptoms of degenerative joint disease.
3. Develop nursing diagnoses for the patient who has undergone joint replacement surgery.

Exercise 1

Writing Activity

15 minutes

1. _____ and _____ are two other names for degenerative joint disease.

2. Which populations are at increased risk for developing degenerative joint disease? Select all that apply.

   _____ Small-framed patients

   _____ Obese patients

   _____ Older patients

   _____ Patients employed in occupations with activities that place joints in stressful positions

   _____ Women of childbearing age

   _____ Patients with diabetes

3. The nurse is reviewing the medical record of a patient suspected of having degenerative joint disease. Which findings are considered consistent with degenerative joint disease? Select all that apply.

   _____ Symmetrical joint discomfort

   _____ Family history of degenerative joint disease

   _____ Changes in joint function noted in hands and hips

   _____ Localized pain and stiffness in affected joints

   _____ Warmth over affected joints

4. What are some management techniques for degenerative joint disease?

5. What is arthroscopy?

6. The nurse is reviewing the laboratory results for the patient with suspected degenerative joint disorder. What results support this potential diagnosis?
   a. Erythrocyte sedimentation rate 25 mm/hr
   b. Rheumatoid factor (RF) 42 units/mL
   c. Serum uric acid level 4 mg/dL
   d. Calcium 10 mg/dL

Exercise 2

Virtual Hospital Activity

45 minutes

- Sign in to work at Pacific View Regional Hospital for Period of Care 1. (*Note:* If you are already in the virtual hospital from a previous exercise, click **Leave the Floor** and then **Restart the Program** to get to the sign-in window.)
- From the Patient List, select Clarence Hughes (Room 404).
- Click **Get Report** and read the Clinical Report.
- Click **Go to Nurses' Station** and then **404** to enter Clarence Hughes' room.
- Read the **Initial Observations**.
- Click **Chart** and then **404** to view Clarence Hughes' chart.
- Click the **History and Physical** tab and review the information given.

1. What signs and symptoms of degenerative joint disease has Clarence Hughes experienced?

2. What other methods of disease management did Clarence Hughes try before he had surgery?

- Click **Return to Room 404**.
- Click **Clinical Alerts** and read the information given.
- Now click **Patient Care** and complete a head-to-toe assessment.

3. _____ Findings from Clarence Hughes' physical assessment warrant physician notification. (True/False)

4. What are the two most important priorities for care at this time?

5. Develop two individualized nursing diagnoses for this patient.

6. Why are these issues most important to the successful management of Clarence Hughes' care?

7. Are there any abnormal findings in the abdominal assessment?

• Click **MAR** and then tab **404** to review Clarence Hughes' record.

8. What medication options are available to manage Clarence Hughes' pain?

- Click **Return to Room 404**.
- Click the **Drug** icon and review the pain medication(s) prescribed for Clarence Hughes.

9. Does Clarence Hughes have any contraindications for the pain medication(s) you identified in question 8?

10. What side effects can be anticipated with administration of the medication(s)?

11. Discuss any safety precautions that may need to be instituted with use of the medication(s).

12. Discuss any special monitoring that will be needed with the administration of the medication(s).

13. What regularly scheduled medication has been ordered to reduce the patient's constipation? What is the mechanism of action for this medication?

14. What prn medications have been ordered to reduce constipation? How do these medications work?

- Click **Return to Room 404**.
- Click **Chart** and then **404** to view Clarence Hughes' chart.
- Click the **Physician's Notes** tab.

15. What are the physician's plans concerning Clarence Hughes' discharge?

- Click the **Consultations** tab.

16. What consultations have been ordered for Clarence Hughes? What is the purpose of these consultations?

- Click the **Patient Education** tab.

17. What are Clarence Hughes' educational needs?

18. List five benefits of early postoperative ambulation.

• Click the **Physician's Orders** tab.

19. After joint replacement surgery, when can the patient anticipate that physical therapy will begin?
    a. Physical therapy will normally begin the day of surgery.
    b. Physical therapy will normally begin 1 to 2 days after surgery.
    c. Physical therapy will begin on a limited basis 3 to 5 days after surgery.
    d. Physical therapy will be prescribed to start at the time of discharge.

20. Generally, patients may begin ambulating _____ to _____ hours after knee replacement surgery.

21. Clarence Hughes' physician has ordered use of a CPM machine. Which term best describes the action of this device?
    a. Passive flexion
    b. Active flexion
    c. Passive extension
    d. Active extension

Postoperative Complications

Reading Assignment: Care of the Surgical Patient (Chapter 2)
Care of the Patient with a Respiratory Disorder (Chapter 9)

Patient: Clarence Hughes, Room 404

Objectives:

1. Identify potential postoperative complications.
2. Recognize clinical manifestations associated with the development of postoperative complications.
3. Review the management/treatment of a postoperative complication involving the respiratory system.

Exercise 1

Writing Activity

15 minutes

1. List several potential postoperative complications.

2. The collapse of lung tissue, which results in the lack of adequate exchange of oxygen and carbon

   dioxide, is known as _____.

3. What is a pulmonary embolism?

4. When assessing the patient for a pulmonary embolism, which manifestation(s) can be anticipated?
   Select all that apply.

   _____   Dull and achy pain

   _____   Pain often described as sharp

   _____   Pain that radiates to the back and neck

   _____   Nonradiating pain

   _____   Dyspnea

   _____   Reduced respiratory rate

   _____   Increased respiratory rate

   _____   Increased pain with inspiration

5. During the initial period after the onset and subsequent diagnosis of a pulmonary embolism, which treatment(s) can be anticipated? Select all that apply.

_____   Oxygen

_____   Oral anticoagulants

_____   Intramuscular antibiotics

_____   Intravenous anticoagulants

_____   Hydration

6. How is a pulmonary embolism managed?

7. What is the prognosis for a patient who develops a pulmonary embolism?

8. Which diagnostic test is considered to be the gold standard for detecting a pulmonary embolism?
   a. Chest radiography
   b. Ventilation perfusion scan
   c. CT scan
   d. Pulmonary angiography

Exercise 2

Virtual Hospital Activity

30 minutes

- Sign in to work at Pacific View Regional Hospital for Period of Care 2. (*Note:* If you are already in the virtual hospital from a previous exercise, click **Leave the Floor** and then **Restart the Program** to get to the sign-in window.)
- From the Patient List, select Clarence Hughes (Room 404).
- Click **Get Report** and read the Clinical Report.

1. Are there any abnormal observations in the report?

2. Review the vital signs recorded in the change-of-shift report. Are they normal?

- Click **Go to Nurses' Station**.
- Click **404** at the bottom of the screen to enter the patient's room.
- Read the **Initial Observations**.
- Click **Clinical Alerts** and read the information provided.

3. Which clinical findings indicate a problem?

- Click **Take Vital Signs**.

4. What are Clarence Hughes' current vital signs?

BP:

T:

HR:

RR:

5. Are any of the above results abnormal? If so, which?

6. What is Clarence Hughes' current oxygen saturation? Is this a normal value? If not, how should it be managed?

- Click **Patient Care** and then **Nurse-Client Interactions**.
- Select and view the video titled **1115: Interventions—Airway**. (*Note:* Check the virtual clock to see whether enough time has elapsed. You can use the fast-forward feature to advance the time by 2-minute intervals if the video is not yet available. Then click again on **Patient Care** and **Nurse-Client Interactions** to refresh the screen.)

7. What behavioral cues being demonstrated by Clarence Hughes indicate a potential health concern?

8. Several nursing interventions are indicated after the onset of Clarence Hughes' breathing problems. Rank the interventions below by matching them in the order in which they need to be completed.

Nursing Intervention	Priority Level
_____ Notify the physician.	a. First
_____ Maintain the airway.	b. Second
_____ Complete a focused assessment.	c. Third
_____ Document care provided.	d. Fourth
_____ Provide education to the family concerning what is taking place.	e. Fifth

- Click **Physical Assessment** and complete a head-to-toe assessment.

9. Are there any significant findings identified in the integumentary assessment?

10. Are there any significant findings identified in the respiratory assessment?

11. Clarence Hughes should be placed in _____ position to facilitate air exchange.

- Click **Chart** and then **404** to view Clarence Hughes' chart.
- Click the **Physician's Orders** tab and review the orders listed for 1120 on Wednesday.

12. What tests and interventions has the physician ordered?

13. The degree of anxiety is often directly tied to the amount of _____ hunger being experienced by the patient.

- Click **Return to Room 404**.
- Click **Patient Care** and then **Nurse-Client Interactions**.
- Select and view the video titled **1135: Change in Patient Condition**. (*Note:* Check the virtual clock to see whether enough time has elapsed. You can use the fast-forward feature to advance the time by 2-minute intervals if the video is not yet available. Then click again on **Patient Care** and **Nurse-Client Interactions** to refresh the screen.)

14. Now that the initial crisis has passed, what are the nurse's priorities concerning the family members?

Exercise 3

Virtual Hospital Activity

15 minutes

- Sign in to work at Pacific View Regional Hospital for Period of Care 3. (*Note:* If you are already in the virtual hospital from the previous exercise, click **Leave the Floor** and then **Restart the Program** to get to the sign-in window.)
- From the Patient List, select Clarence Hughes (Room 404).
- Click **Get Report** and read the report.

1. Give the results for each of the tests listed below.

    a. Arterial blood gas:

    b. Chest x-ray:

    c. Ventilation perfusion scan:

    d. Doppler study:

- Click **Go to Nurses' Station**.
- Click **404** at the bottom of the screen to enter Clarence Hughes' room.
- Read the **Initial Observations**.
- Click and review the **Clinical Alerts**.

2. What changes are noted in the patient's demeanor and clinical manifestations?

• Click **Take Vital Signs** and review the results.

3. What is the significance of the increasing SpO$_2$ level?

• Click **Chart** and then **404** to review Clarence Hughes' chart.
• Click the **Physician's Orders** tab and review the information given.

4. What medication has been ordered to manage Clarence Hughes' condition? Describe the administration of this medication.

5. What is the method of action and the purpose for the administration of this medication?

6. What is the classification of this medication?

7. During therapy with the medication identified in question 4, which laboratory test is most important to monitor?
   a. PTT
   b. Hgb
   c. Hct
   d. WBC
   e. ESR

8. Once the intravenous anticoagulant therapy has been tapered off, Clarence Hughes can anticipate continuing on oral therapy for a period of:
   a. 3 months.
   b. 6 months.
   c. 9 months.
   d. 1 year.
   e. 18 months.

LESSON **6**

Care of the Patient with Pneumonia

Reading Assignment: Care of the Patient with a Respiratory Disorder (Chapter 9)

Patient: Patricia Newman, Room 406

Objectives:

1. Define pneumonia.
2. Identify the potential causes of pneumonia.
3. Identify the populations at risk for pneumonia.
4. Discuss nursing care for the patient with pneumonia.

Exercise 1

Writing Activity

30 minutes

1. What is pneumonia?

2. Infants and _____ are most susceptible to pneumonia.

3. What factors may increase susceptibility to pneumonia?

4. Which factors may contribute to the development of pneumonia? Select all that apply.

   _____ Overuse of steroid medications

   _____ Infection

   _____ Hyperventilation

   _____ Inadequate ventilation

   _____ Aspiration

   _____ Poor nutritional habits

5. Match the columns below to show the correct order of pathologic occurrences associated with the development of pneumonia.

Disease Process	Order of Occurrence
_____ The respiratory tract develops inflammation and localized edema.	a. First
	b. Second
_____ The exchange of oxygen and carbon dioxide becomes increasingly reduced.	c. Third
_____ Secretions begin to accumulate and are not able to be moved by the cilia in the lungs.	d. Fourth
_____ Retained secretions become infected.	

6. When caring for a patient diagnosed with pneumonia, which nursing interventions are appropriate? Select all that apply.

_____ Keep patient on complete bedrest.

_____ Encourage deep breathing and coughing activities.

_____ Initiate exercise training.

_____ Provide patient education aimed at reducing the spread of infection.

_____ Restrict protein intake.

_____ Monitor vital signs and pulmonary status.

_____ Provide information concerning the prescribed medication therapy.

_____ Encourage fluid intake if not contraindicated by patient's coexisting conditions.

7. What is the typical prognosis for a patient with pneumonia?

8. When assisting the patient with pneumonia to plan meals, which dietary recommendation should be implemented?
   a. Three large balanced meals each day will be best to provide the needed nutrients.
   b. The diet should include at least 3000 calories per day.
   c. Protein and sodium are indicated.
   d. The diet should consist of at least 1500 calories each day.

9. What is the purpose of the above dietary intervention?

10. The patient with pneumonia should consume at least _____ of fluid per day unless contra-indicated by other medical conditions.

Exercise 2

Virtual Hospital Activity

30 minutes

- Sign in to work at Pacific View Regional Hospital for Period of Care 1. (*Note:* If you are already in the virtual hospital from a previous exercise, click **Leave the Floor** and then **Restart the Program** to get to the sign-in window.)
- From the Patient List, select Patricia Newman (Room 406).
- Click **Get Report** and read the Clinical Report.
- Click **Go to Nurses' Station**.
- Click **Chart** and then **406** to view Patricia Newman's chart.
- Click the **Emergency Department** tab and review the information given.

1. What were the findings of the Initial Assessment in the emergency department?

2. Discuss any abnormal findings in her respiratory system assessment.

3. Find the vital sign results on the ED record and discuss the significance of these findings.

4. What are the primary and secondary admitting diagnoses?

5. Listed below are laboratory tests ordered for Patricia Newman while in the emergency department. Match each laboratory test with its reason for being ordered.

Laboratory Test	**Reason It Was Ordered**
_____ Sputum gram stain	a. To provide information about the potential presence of infection and the body's response
_____ Arterial blood gases	b. To identify specific pathogens in a specimen
_____ Complete blood count	c. To identify the specific pathogens and determine which medications therapies will be most effective
_____ Culture and sensitivity	d. To identify the presence and degree of inflammation in the body
_____ Erythrocyte sedimentation rate	e. To definitely evaluate the oxygen levels in the body

6. Patricia Newman's physician has ordered a chest x-ray. What is the rationale for ordering this test?

- Click **Return to Nurses' Station**.
- Click **406** at the bottom of the screen and review the **Initial Observations**.

7. Discuss the significance of the oxygen saturation and the patient's removal of the nasal cannula.

- Click **Return to Room 406**.
- Click **Take Vital Signs** and review the results provided.

8. What are the patient's current vital signs, including oxygen saturation and pain level?

BP:

SpO_2:

T:

HR:

RR:

Pain:

9. Review Patricia Newman's vital signs listed above. What is the significance of these findings?

- Click **Patient Care** and complete a head-to-toe assessment.

10. What assessment findings support the admitting diagnosis of pneumonia?

- Click **MAR** and then tab **406** to review the medications ordered for Patricia Newman.

11. The following drugs have been ordered to manage Patricia Newman's pneumonia. Match each drug with its correct classification.

Drug	Classification
_____ Acetaminophen	a. Antipyretic
_____ Cefotan	b. Antiinflammatory
_____ Ipratropium	c. Antibiotic
	d. Bronchodilator
	e. Corticosteroid

- Click **Return to Room 406**.
- Click **Chart** and then **406** to view Patricia Newman's chart.
- Click the **Laboratory Reports** tab and review the information given.

12. Patricia Newman had arterial blood gases drawn on Wednesday. Review her results below. Which are within normal limits? Select all that apply.

_____ pH: 7.33

_____ PaO_2: 70 mm Hg

_____ $PaCO_2$: 47 mm Hg

13. Review Patricia Newman's arterial gas pH level of 7.33. What is this level most reflective of?
    a. Acidity
    b. Alkalinity

14. With consideration to the pH, PO_2, and PCO_2 levels, which interpretation of the arterial blood gases is most likely?
    a. Metabolic acidosis
    b. Metabolic alkalosis
    c. Respiratory acidosis
    d. Respiratory alkalosis

15. Discuss the significance of the culture and sensitivity test results.

16. Review and discuss the findings of the complete blood count test.

- Click the **Diagnostic Reports** tab and review the report.

17. Review the chest x-ray. What findings are consistent with the diagnosis of pneumonia?

18. Which clinical manifestations will reflect positive impact of treatments?

19. _____ Patricia Newman should take the pneumococcal vaccine. (True/False)

Care of the Patient Experiencing Comorbid Conditions (Musculoskeletal and Respiratory)

Reading Assignment: Care of the Patient with a Musculoskeletal Disorder (Chapter 4)

Care of the Patient with a Cardiovascular or a Peripheral Vascular Disorder (Chapter 8)

Care of the Patient with a Respiratory Disorder (Chapter 9)

Patient: Patricia Newman, Room 406

Objectives:

1. Identify significant findings in a patient's medical history.
2. Identify significant findings in a patient's social history.
3. Discuss the pathophysiology, risk factors, and management of hypertension.
4. Discuss the pathophysiology, risk factors, and management of osteoporosis.
5. Discuss the pathophysiology, risk factors, and management of emphysema.
6. Identify important issues in caring for the patient with comorbid conditions.

Exercise 1

Writing Activity

30 minutes

1. Hypertension is classified by which criteria?
   a. Blood pressure of 130/80 mm Hg or above on one occasion.
   b. Blood pressure of 140/90 mm Hg or above on two occasions.
   c. Sustained blood pressure readings above 140/85 mm Hg.
   d. Sustained blood pressure reading of 140/80 on three occasions.

2. Which risk factors are associated with hypertension? Select all that apply.

   _____ Obesity

   _____ Genetic factors

   _____ Sedentary lifestyle

   _____ Diabetes

   _____ Asthma

   _____ Increased sodium intake

   _____ Excessive alcohol ingestion

3. List three medical management options for the treatment of hypertension.

4. What is emphysema?

LESSON 7—CARE OF THE PATIENT EXPERIENCING COMORBID CONDITIONS **89**

5. Which are risk factors associated with emphysema? Select all that apply.

_____ Family history

_____ History of diabetes

_____ Cigarette use

_____ Environmental exposure to dust

_____ Having worked as a grain bin operator

6. Which are clinical manifestations associated with emphysema? Select all that apply.

_____ Dyspnea with exertion

_____ Hypertension

_____ Tachypnea

_____ Bradypnea

_____ Tachycardia

_____ Bradycardia

_____ Use of accessory muscles with breathing

_____ Weight gain

_____ Barrel-chested appearance

_____ Clubbing of fingers

7. What is the usual prognosis for a patient diagnosed with emphysema?

8. Osteoporosis is a disease characterized by the reduction in _____.

9. Which populations are at high risk for the development of osteoporosis? Select all that apply.

    _____ Women

    _____ Large-framed individuals

    _____ Smokers

    _____ Those with sedentary lifestyles

    _____ People taking supplements to increase calcium intake

    _____ Users of steroids

    _____ Immobilized individuals

    _____ Postmenopausal women

    _____ African Americans

10. What areas of the body are most affected by osteoporosis?

11. A nurse is planning care for a patient suspected of having osteoporosis. Which tests may be used to confirm the diagnosis? Select all that apply.

    _____ Chest x-ray

    _____ CBC

    _____ Bone mineral density test

    _____ Thyroid function tests

    _____ Liver function test

    _____ EMG

12. List several clinical manifestations associated with osteoporosis.

13. When planning the care of a patient diagnosed with osteoporosis, the nurse knows that which interventions may be included? Select all that apply.

_____ Exercise

_____ Restricted levels of activity

_____ Increased calcium intake/supplements

_____ Estrogen therapy

_____ Reduced protein intake

14. When planning a diet high in calcium, which foods should be included?
    a. Yellow vegetables
    b. Tomatoes
    c. Dates and legumes
    d. Green leafy vegetables

Exercise 2

Virtual Hospital Activity

45 minutes

- Sign in to work at Pacific View Regional Hospital for Period of Care 3. (*Note:* If you are already in the virtual hospital from a previous exercise, click **Leave the Floor** and then **Restart the Program** to get to the sign-In window.)
- From the Patient List, select Patricia Newman (Room 406).
- Click **Go to Nurses' Station**.
- Click **Chart** and then click **406**.
- Click the **History and Physical** tab and review the information provided.

1. What significant medical issues are in Patricia Newman's medical history?

2. The coexistence of osteoporosis, emphysema, and hypertension presents what unique problems for Patricia Newman?

3. Does the patient have any surgeries in her medical history?

4. Describe Patricia Newman's social history.

• Still in Patricia Newman's chart, click the **Nursing Admission** tab and review the information given.
• Click the **Laboratory Reports** tab and review the test results.

5. What factors in Patricia Newman's history are related to a diagnosis of emphysema?

6. How is her recurring history of pneumonia related to her emphysema?

7. Review Patricia Newman's medical history. Which findings are associated with her diagnosis of osteoporosis? Select all that apply.

_____ Age

_____ Gender

_____ Sedentary lifestyle

_____ Tobacco use

_____ Underweight status

8. Patricia Newman has which type of pneumonia?
   a. Bacterial pneumonia
   b. Viral pneumonia
   c. Aspiration pneumonia

- Click **Return to Nurses' Station**.
- Click **406** at the bottom of the screen to go to Patricia Newman's room.
- Click **Take Vital Signs** and review the results.
- Next, click **Patient Care** and perform a focused physical assessment.

9. What vital signs and/or assessment findings are consistent with a diagnosis of pneumonia?

- Now click **MAR**.
- Click tab **406** to view the medications ordered for Patricia Newman.

10. What medications have been prescribed to manage Patricia Newman's hypertension?

11. Describe the mode of action for each of the medications that you identified in question 10.

12. When you are planning care for the patient being treated with the above medications, which laboratory test must be monitored?
    a. Serum sodium levels
    b. Serum potassium levels
    c. Erythrocyte sedimentation rate
    d. Complete blood count results

13. What medications have been ordered to manage Patricia Newman's emphysema?

14. What medication has been prescribed to manage Patricia Newman's osteoporosis?

15. After reviewing Patricia Newman's medical history, the nurse recognizes that which is the appropriate amount of calcium to be included in her daily diet?
    a. 750 mg
    b. 1000 mg
    c. 1250 mg
    d. 1500 mg

16. Which nursing implications are indicated when administering the medication ordered to manage osteoporosis? Select all that apply.

    _____   Administer medication 15 to 30 minutes before eating.

    _____   Administer medication with juice to improve absorption.

    _____   Administer medication 30 to 60 minutes after eating.

    _____   Monitor blood pressure.

    _____   Administer with foods high in fiber.

Prioritizing Care for the Patient with a Pulmonary Disorder

Reading Assignment: Care of the Patient with a Respiratory Disorder (Chapter 9)

Patient: Patricia Newman, Room 406

Objectives:

1. Review the diagnostic tests performed on the patient with emphysema.
2. Identify the primary patient education goals for the patient experiencing a pulmonary disorder.
3. Discuss the appropriate service consultations for a patient experiencing a pulmonary disorder.
4. Determine the impact of personal/social factors in the patient's recovery period.
5. Develop priorities for the patient during hospitalization and in preparation for discharge.

Exercise 1

Writing Activity

30 minutes

1. Which are characteristics associated with emphysema? Select all that apply.

    _____ Emphysema affects both men and women.

    _____ Emphysema symptoms typically begin to manifest while the patient is in the mid- to late 30s.

    _____ The disorder is characterized by changes in the alveolar walls and capillaries.

    _____ Disability often results in patients diagnosed with emphysema between ages 50 and 60 years.

    _____ Heredity may play a role in the development of emphysema.

2. When diagnostic tests are ordered to confirm the presence of emphysema, which tests may be anticipated? Select all that apply.

    _____ Thoracentesis

    _____ Arterial blood gases

    _____ Complete blood cell count

    _____ Chest x-ray

    _____ Bronchoscopy

    _____ Pulse oximetry

3. When caring for a patient diagnosed with emphysema, the nurse should anticipate which result for a pulmonary function test?
   a. Reduced residual volume
   b. Reduced airway resistance
   c. Increased ventilatory response
   d. Increased residual volume

4. The complete blood cell count will reflect which result(s) in a patient diagnosed with emphysema?
   a. Reduced erythrocyte count
   b. Elevated erythrocyte count
   c. Elevated erythrocyte count and reduced hemoglobin
   d. Reduced erythrocyte count and elevated hemoglobin

5. In the patient who is experiencing emphysema, which result best reflects the anticipated pulmonary function tests?
   a. Increased PaO_2
   b. Decreased PaO_2
   c. Reduced residual volume
   d. Increased total lung capacity

6. Describe the disease process associated with emphysema.

7. Indicate whether each statement is true or false.

   a. _____   An inherited form of emphysema is due to an oversecretion of a liver protein
                         known as ATT.

   b. _____   Hypercapnia does not develop until the later stages of emphysema.

8. Discuss the use of exercise in the care and management of the patient diagnosed with emphysema.

9. _____ is an abnormal cardiac condition characterized by hypertrophy of the
   right ventricle of the heart due to hypertension of the pulmonary circulation.

10. What are the management options for the patient with emphysema?

Exercise 2

Virtual Hospital Activity

30 minutes

- Sign in to work at Pacific View Regional Hospital for Period of Care 3. (*Note:* If you are already in the virtual hospital from a previous exercise, click **Leave the Floor** and then **Restart the Program** to get to the sign-in window.)
- From the Patient List, select Patricia Newman (Room 406).
- Click **Get Report** and read the Clinical Report.
- Click **Go to Nurses' Station**.
- Click **406** at the bottom of the screen. Read the **Initial Observations**.
- Click **Patient Care** and then **Nurse-Client Interactions**.
- Select and view the video titled **1500: Discharge Planning**. (*Note:* Check the virtual clock to see whether enough time has elapsed. You can use the fast-forward feature to advance the time by 2-minute intervals if the video is not yet available. Then click again on **Patient Care** and **Nurse-Client Interactions** to refresh the screen.)

1. Discuss Patricia Newman's demeanor during the video interaction.

2. What appear to be the patient's biggest concerns during this interaction?

- Click **Physical Assessment** and complete a head-to-toe assessment.

3. What evidence suggests that Patricia Newman's condition is improving?

4. Are there any assessment findings that could potentially have a negative implication for Patricia Newman's discharge to home? If so, explain.

5. When preparing to discharge Patricia Newman, the nurse will need to review the patient's understanding of the correct use of the metered inhaler. Which observation would indicate the need for additional teaching?
   a. Patricia Newman rinses her mouth out with water immediately after inhalation.
   b. Patricia Newman waits 1 minute between inhaling her first and her second dose.
   c. Patricia Newman shakes the medicine container before use.
   d. Patricia Newman holds her breath as long as she can after administering the medication.

6. As you develop Patricia Newman's plan of care, which are priorities at this time? Select all that apply.

   _____ Dietary counseling

   _____ Preparation for discharge

   _____ Referrals for smoking cessation programs

   _____ Requesting a consultation with physical therapy

   _____ Requesting a consultation with social services

7. Develop three nursing diagnoses for Patricia Newman.

- Click **Chart** and then **406** to view Patricia Newman's chart.
- Click the **Nursing Admission** tab and review the information given.

8. Identify Patricia Newman's social concerns.

9. Which statement accurately reflects an aspect of Patricia Newman's needs?
   a. She has numerous friends and family members available to provide assistance.
   b. She appears self-sufficient and needs little outside help.
   c. She is somewhat socially isolated.
   d. Her significant other will be available as needed for assistance after discharge.

10. Discuss the implications of these social concerns on the nurse's plan of care for Patricia Newman.

• Click the **Patient Education** tab and review the information given.

11. Which dietary recommendations should be included in Patricia Newman's patient teaching? Select all that apply.

   _____ Avoid resting before eating.

   _____ Recommended oral fluid intake should be 1 to 2 L/day.

   _____ 5 to 6 meals per day are recommended.

   _____ Meals should be high in calories.

   _____ Meals should be low in fiber.

   _____ Moderate protein is recommended.

12. As Patricia Newman prepares to go home, which are educational goals for her discharge? Select all that apply.

   _____ Correct use of MDI and peak flow meter

   _____ Understanding the rationale for and performance of pursed-lip breathing and effective cough technique

   _____ The need to be sedentary to avoid further complications

   _____ Understanding of and compliance with her prescribed medication therapy

   _____ Compliance with progressive activity/exercise goals

13. Considering Patricia Newman's social and financial history, which goals may be a challenge for her to meet?

14. When discussing immunization recommendations with Patricia Newman, what information should be included?
    a. The pneumonia vaccine is recommended every 2 years.
    b. The pneumonia vaccine cannot be taken during the same season as the influenza vaccine.
    c. The influenza vaccine is recommended each year.
    d. The influenza vaccine and the pneumonia vaccine are recommended each year.

• Click the **Physician's Orders** tab.

15. What consultations have been ordered for Patricia Newman during this hospitalization?

9

Care of the Patient Experiencing Exacerbation of an Asthmatic Condition

Reading Assignment: Care of the Patient with a Respiratory Disorder (Chapter 9)

Patient: Jacquline Catanazaro, Room 402

Objectives:

1. Define asthma.
2. Identify factors that contribute to an asthmatic episode.
3. Report assessment findings consistent with an exacerbation of asthma.
4. Discuss the impact of emotional distress on the respiratory system.

Exercise 1

Writing Activity

15 minutes

1. What is asthma?

2. Which statement concerning the mechanisms of asthma is true?
   a. Air tubes narrow as a result of swollen tissues and excessive mucus production.
   b. Edema of the respiratory mucosa and excessive mucus production occur, thus obstructing airways.
   c. The walls of the alveoli are torn and cannot be repaired.
   d. The bronchioles are scarred and unable to expand.

3. List the clinical manifestations of mild asthma.

4. List the signs and symptoms associated with an acute asthmatic attack.

5. Which events can trigger an asthmatic episode? Select all that apply.

    _____ Hormone levels

    _____ Mental and physical fatigue

    _____ Emotional factors

    _____ Environmental exposures

    _____ Electrolyte imbalances

6. When an asthmatic condition is suspected, which diagnostic tests will confirm a diagnosis? Select all that apply.

    _____ Complete blood count

    _____ Serum electrolyte levels

    _____ Arterial blood gas

    _____ Pulmonary function tests

    _____ Sputum cultures

7. A _____ should be obtained to rule out a secondary infection.

8. When a patient is experiencing an asthma attack, a complete blood cell count will show an elevation in which blood cell type?
   a. Eosinophils
   b. Platelets
   c. Red blood cells
   d. Monocytes

9. Which is correct concerning the impact of oxygen saturation levels on the body's functioning?
   a. Saturation rates of 95% to 100% are needed to replenish oxygen in the plasma.
   b. Saturation rates below 90% affect the ability of hemoglobin to feed oxygen to the plasma.
   c. Saturation levels below 70% are considered life-threatening.
   d. Saturation levels below 85% warrant contacting the physician.

Exercise 2

Virtual Hospital Activity

45 minutes

- Sign in to work at Pacific View Regional Hospital for Period of Care 1. (*Note:* If you are already in the virtual hospital from a previous exercise, click **Leave the Floor** and then **Restart the Program** to get to the sign-in window.)
- From the Patient List, select Jacquline Catanazaro (Room 402).
- Click **Get Report** and read the Clinical Report.
- Click **Go to Nurses' Station**.
- Click **Chart** and then **402** to view Jacquline Catanazaro's chart.
- Click the **Emergency Department** tab and review the information given.

1. Review the admitting vital signs. What is the significance of the findings?

2. What is the primary admitting diagnosis?

- Click **Return to Nurses' Station** and then **402** at the bottom of the screen.
- Read the **Initial Observations**.
- Click **Take Vital Signs** and review the results.
- Click **Clinical Alerts** and read the report.

3. Jacquline Catanazaro is demonstrating extreme agitation. What is the impact of this on her health status?

4. When preparing to perform a pulse oximeter reading on Jacquline Catanazaro, which sites would be appropriate for this test? Select all that apply.

_____ Ear lobe

_____ Bridge of the nose

_____ Tip of the nose

_____ Finger

_____ Toe

5. _____ When using the pulse oximeter, the probe should be placed over a pulsating vascular bed. (True/False)

- Click **Patient Care** and then **Nurse-Client Interactions**.
- Select and view the video titled **0730: Intervention—Airway**. (*Note:* Check the virtual clock to see whether enough time has elapsed. You can use the fast-forward feature to advance the time by 2-minute intervals if the video is not yet available. Then click again on **Patient Care** and **Nurse-Client Interactions** to refresh the screen.)

6. Jacquline Catanazaro is experiencing an acute asthma attack. What has been planned to manage the onset of this attack?

7. What will the arterial blood gases determine?

- Click **Physical Assessment** and complete a head-to-toe assessment.

8. What respiratory system findings in Jacquline Catanazaro's assessment are consistent with an exacerbation of asthma?

9. Jacquline Catanazaro's lung assessment reveals the presence of wheezes. Which description is consistent with wheezes?
   a. Heard most frequently with inspiration
   b. Caused by air movement through narrowed bronchioles
   c. Caused by fluid, mucus, or pus in the small airways and alveoli
   d. Dry, creaking, grating, low-pitched sounds heard during inspiration and expiration

10. Jacquline Catanazaro's lung assessment reveals the presence of crackles. Which description is consistent with crackles?
    a. Bubbling sounds that are similar to the sound produced when strands of hair are rubbed between the fingers
    b. Caused by inflammation of the respiratory tree
    c. Loud machine-like sounds heard over the anterior chest wall
    d. High-pitched musical sounds heard with inspiration or expiration

11. Are there any other significant system findings?

- Click **Chart** and then **402** to view Jacquline Catanazaro's chart.
- Click the **Physician's Orders** tab and note the admission orders for Monday at 1600.
- Click **Return to Room 402** and then click the **Drug** icon at the bottom of the screen.
- Review the information for the drugs that have been prescribed for Jacquline Catanazaro.

12. What are the doses and routes of administration for each of the medications ordered to manage Jacquline Catanazaro's respiratory condition?

    a. Beclomethasone:

    b. Albuterol:

    c. Ipratropium bromide:

13. Below, match each prescribed medication with its correct mode of action.

Medication	Mode of Action
_____ Beclomethasone	a. Relief of bronchospasms
_____ Albuterol	b. Reduction of bronchial inflammation
_____ Ipratropium bromide	c. Control of secretions

14. When providing patient education concerning the use of beclomethasone, which should be included in the list of potential side effects associated with the medication? Select all that apply.

_____ Throat irritation

_____ Cough

_____ Nausea

_____ Nasal dryness

_____ Skin rash

• Click **Return to Room 402**.
• Click **Chart** and then **402**.
• Click the **Physician's Orders** tab and review the orders for Monday at 1600.

15. What tests and/or assessments will be used to monitor Jacquline Catanazaro's respiratory status?

• Click **Return to Room 402**.
• Click **Patient Care** and then **Nurse-Client Interactions**.
• Select and view the video titled **0800: Managing Altered Perceptions**. (*Note:* Check the virtual clock to see whether enough time has elapsed. You can use the fast-forward feature to advance the time by 2-minute intervals if the video is not yet available. Then click again on **Patient Care** and **Nurse-Client Interactions** to refresh the screen.)

16. What medication has been ordered for Jacquline Catanazaro?

17. What are the classification and mode of action for this medication?

18. List several clinical manifestations that would indicate improvement in Jacquline Catanazaro's condition.

10

Developing a Plan of Care for the Asthmatic Patient with Psychological Complications

Reading Assignment: Care of the Patient with a Respiratory Disorder (Chapter 9)

Patient: Jacquline Catanazaro, Room 402

Objectives:

1. Evaluate the impact of the patient's social history on anticipated compliance after discharge.
2. Identify the elements to be incorporated into the teaching plan in preparation for discharge.
3. Develop nursing diagnoses for the patient experiencing coexisting psychological and physiologic conditions.

Exercise 1

Writing Activity

15 minutes

1. _____ is a severe asthmatic attack that fails to respond to the normal treatment plan.

2. What extrinsic factors are associated with an asthmatic attack? Select all that apply.

   _____ Infection

   _____ Dust

   _____ Pollen

   _____ Exercise

   _____ Foods

3. When caring for the patient with asthma, it is imperative for the nurse to recognize that which manifestations are associated with hypoxia? Select all that apply.

   _____ Restlessness

   _____ Tachycardia

   _____ Fever

   _____ Bradycardia

   _____ Confusion

4. What is the prognosis for asthma?

5. Match the columns below to show which characteristics are related to each condition. Note that conditions may be used more than one time.

Characteristic	Condition
_____ Airflow on exhalation is slowed or stopped by overinflated alveoli.	a. Chronic bronchitis
_____ Excessive amounts of mucus in the airways obstructs airways.	b. Asthma
_____ Exposure to irritants cause the bronchial smooth muscles to constrict.	c. Emphysema
_____ Disease process results in impaired ciliary function.	

6. Which range is considered acceptable for a therapeutic level of theophylline?
   a. 35 to 45 mcg/mL
   b. Less than 4 mcg/mL
   c. 10 to 20 mcg/mL
   d. Greater than 50 mcg/mL

7. Match each drug with its correct classification.

Drug	Classification
_____ Serevent	a. Corticosteroid
_____ Flovent	b. Long-acting beta receptor agonist
_____ Adrenalin	c. Short-acting beta receptor agonist
_____ Proventil	d. Bronchodilator

Exercise 2

Virtual Hospital Activity

45 minutes

- Sign in to work at Pacific View Regional Hospital for Period of Care 2. (*Note:* If you are already in the Virtual Hospital from a previous exercise, click **Leave the Floor** and then **Restart the Program** to get to the sign-in window.)
- From the Patient List, select Jacquline Catanazaro (Room 402).
- Click **Get Report** and read the Clinical Report.

1. Describe the psychological behaviors documented in the two change-of-shift reports.

2. How do these psychological behaviors affect Jacquline Catanazaro's condition?

- Click **Go to Nurses' Station** and then **402**.
- Read the **Initial Observations**.
- Click **Take Vital Signs** and review the findings.
- Click **Patient Care** and complete a head-to-toe assessment.
- Next, click **Nurse-Client Interactions**.
- Select and view the video titled **1115: Assessment—Readiness to Learn**. (*Note:* Check the virtual clock to see whether enough time has elapsed. You can use the fast-forward feature to advance the time by 2-minute intervals if the video is not yet available. Then click again on **Patient Care** and **Nurse-Client Interactions** to refresh the screen.)

3. What is the focus of the video interaction?

4. Do social supports appear to be available for Jacquline Catanazaro?

5. What are the priorities of care associated with Jacquline Catanazaro's psychosocial needs?

6. What are the priorities of care associated with Jacquline Catanazaro's physiologic needs?

• Click **Chart** and then **402** to view Jacquline Catanazaro's chart.
• Click the **History and Physical** tab and review the information given.

7. List some significant issues identified in Jacquline Catanazaro's medical history.

8. List several significant issues identified in Jacquline Catanazaro's social history.

9. Describe the interrelationships among the medical and social elements in Jacquline Catanazaro's history.

10. What factors in Jacquline Catanazaro's medical history will significantly affect her discharge?

11. How does Jacquline Catanazaro's mental health affect her physical health?

- Still in the patient's chart, click the **Consultations** tab and review the information given.

12. Discuss the plan identified in the Psychiatric Consult report.

- Click the **Patient Education** tab and review the education goals listed.

13. What educational goals are identified?

14. Who should be included in the teaching plan for Jacquline Catanazaro?

15. When preparing for discharge, the nurse will need to ensure that Jacquline Catanazaro understands the medications that have been prescribed. What information should be included concerning the prescribed corticosteroids?
    a. Take with food to minimize stomach upset.
    b. Avoid taking with milk.
    c. Do not use OTC cold preparations.
    d. Take medications immediately upon awakening each morning.

16. When reviewing potential side effects of the prescribed medications, which reactions is associated with ipratropium and should be reported to the physician?
    a. Acute eye pain
    b. Dry mouth
    c. Cough
    d. Nasal irritation

17. Develop two nursing diagnoses for the patient at this point in her care.

LESSON **11**

Care and Treatment of the Patient with Complications of Cancer

Reading Assignment: Care of the Patient with Cancer (Chapter 17)

Patient: Pablo Rodriguez, Room 405

Objectives:

1. Discuss complications associated with cancer.
2. Discuss the management of the patient experiencing dehydration secondary to chemotherapy.
3. Prioritize the problems of the patient experiencing complications of cancer.
4. Evaluate abnormal laboratory findings.

Exercise 1

Virtual Hospital Activity

15 minutes

- Sign in to work at Pacific View Regional Hospital for Period of Care 2. (*Note:* If you are already in the virtual hospital from a previous exercise, click **Leave the Floor** and then **Restart the Program** to get to the sign-in window.)
- From the Patient List, select Pablo Rodriguez (Room 405).
- Click **Get Report** and read the Clinical Report.
- Click **Go to Nurses' Station**.
- Click **Chart** and then **405** to view Pablo Rodriguez's chart.
- Click the **Emergency Department** tab and review the information given.

1. What are the four priorities identified in the change-of-shift report?

2. Why was Pablo Rodriguez admitted to the hospital?

3. What has caused this condition?

4. What findings support this diagnosis?

5. How was his condition initially managed in the emergency department?

6. What types of interventions (nursing and medical) may be implemented to manage his care?

7. What should be monitored to determine the degree of dehydration?

8. What are the primary goals for this hospitalization?

• Click the **History and Physical** tab and read the report.

9. List the impressions identified in the History and Physical.

Exercise 2

Virtual Hospital Activity

30 minutes

- Sign in to work at Pacific View Regional Hospital for Period of Care 2. (*Note:* If you are already in the virtual hospital from a previous exercise, click **Leave the Floor** and then **Restart the Program** to get to the sign-in window.)
- From the Patient List, select Pablo Rodriguez (Room 405).
- Click **Go to Nurses' Station**.
- Click **405** at the bottom of the screen to enter Pablo Rodriguez's room.
- Click **Take Vital Signs** and then **Clinical Alerts** and review the information given.
- Read the **Initial Observations** and read the notes.
- Click **Patient Care** and complete a head-to-toe assessment.

  1. What current assessment findings support the diagnosis of dehydration?

- Click **Chart** and then **405** to view Pablo Rodriguez's chart.
- Click the **Physician's Orders** tab and review the orders since Tuesday at 2300.

  2. Which medications have been ordered to manage Pablo Rodriguez's nausea?

- Click **Return to Room 405** and then click the **Drug** icon at the bottom of the screen.
- Review the medications you identified in the previous question.

  3. To which drug classification does ondansetron hydrochloride belong?

4. What side effects of ondansetron could be problematic, considering Pablo Rodriguez's health concerns?

5. What is metoclopramide's mechanism of action?

- Click **Return to Room 405**.
- Once again, click **Chart** and then **405**.
- This time, click the **Laboratory Reports** tab and review the report given.

6. Review and discuss any significant findings in the CBC results.

7. Consider the clinical presentation of Pablo Rodriguez. Which manifestations may be attributed to his complete blood cell test results? Select all that apply.

_____ Nausea

_____ Vomiting

_____ Weaknesses

_____ Fatigue

_____ Reduced skin turgor

8. Are there any significant findings in the electrolyte profile?

9. Identify two nursing diagnoses related to Pablo Rodriguez's primary admitting diagnosis.

Exercise 3

Virtual Hospital Activity

30 minutes

- Sign in to work at Pacific View Regional Hospital for Period of Care 2. (*Note:* If you are already in the virtual hospital from a previous exercise, click **Leave the Floor** and then **Restart the Program** to get to the sign-in window.)
- From the Patient List, select Pablo Rodriguez (Room 405).
- Click **Get Report** and read the Clinical Report.
- Click **Go to Nurses' Station** and then **405** at the bottom of the screen to enter Pablo Rodriguez's room.
- Click **Take Vital Signs** and review the information given.

1. How does Pablo Rodriguez rate his pain?

- Click **MAR** and then tab **405** to review the medications ordered for Pablo Rodriguez.

2. What medications have been ordered to manage Pablo Rodriguez's pain?

3. What is the advantage of this type of dosing?

4. List some opioids that may be prescribed to manage the pain associated with advanced cancer.

5. When administering opioids to manage Pablo Rodriguez's pain, the nurse must understand that which manifestations are common side effects associated with their use? Select all that apply.

_____ Diarrhea

_____ Constipation

_____ Bradycardia

_____ Rash

_____ Respiratory depression

_____ Hyperthermia

_____ Vomiting

6. List several nonopioid medications that can be administered to reduce mild to moderate pain associated with cancer.

7. Discuss medication scheduling techniques that effectively manage pain.

8. As previously stated, Pablo Rodriguez has been experiencing anxiety. Discuss the relationship between pain and anxiety.

9. In addition to medication therapy, what other interventions may be used to manage pain?

10. What factors may influence a patient's perception of and/or reaction to pain?

- Click **Return to Room 405**.
- Click **Patient Care** and then **Nurse-Client Interactions**.
- Select and view the video titled **1130: Family Interaction**. (*Note:* Check the virtual clock to see whether enough time has elapsed. You can use the fast-forward feature to advance the time by 2-minute intervals if the video is not yet available. Then click again on **Patient Care** and **Nurse-Client Interactions** to refresh the screen.)

11. What is the underlying message Pablo Rodriguez is attempting to communicate to his daughter?
    a. He is too tired to attend her wedding.
    b. The enema has made him feel better.
    c. He is ready to give in to the disease and die.
    d. The enema has caused him pain.

12. Does the response by Pablo Rodriguez's daughter indicate a readiness to accept her father's condition?

13. _____ Pablo Rodriguez will be allowed to make the decision to forgo further treatment without the approval of his immediate family. (True/False)

14. Identify referrals that may be beneficial for Pablo Rodriguez and his family at this time.

12

Care and Treatment of the Patient with Cancer

Reading Assignment: Care of the Patient with Cancer (Chapter 17)

Patient: Pablo Rodriguez, Room 405

Objectives:

1. Identify the physiologic changes associated with the diagnosis of cancer.
2. List risk factors for the development of cancer.
3. Identify the tests that may be used to diagnose cancer.
4. Define metastasis.

Exercise 1

Writing Activity

30 minutes

1. Which foods have been shown to reduce the risk for cancer? Select all that apply.

   _____ Broccoli

   _____ Lettuce

   _____ Bananas

   _____ Carrots

   _____ Grapefruit

   _____ Tomatoes

2. Consuming at least _____ servings of fruits and vegetables per day has been shown to reduce the risk for cancer.

3. _____ The risk for the development of lung cancer is similar among users of smokeless tobacco and cigarette smokers. (True/False)

4. A variety of diagnostic tests may be utilized to assess for potential malignancies. Match each diagnostic test with its correct description.

Diagnostic Test	Description
_____ Computed tomography	a. Noninvasive, high-frequency sound waves are used to examine external body structures.
_____ Radioisotope studies	b. A computer is used to process radiofrequency energy waves to assess spinal lesions, as well as cardiovascular and soft tissue abnormalities.
_____ Ultrasound testing	c. Radiographs and computed scanning are used to provide images of structures at differing angles.
_____ Magnetic resonance imaging	d. A substance is injected or ingested; then the uptake is evaluated to identify areas of concern.

5. Which characteristics are associated with benign growths? Select all that apply.

_____ Rapid growth

_____ Smooth and well-defined

_____ Immobile when palpated

_____ Often recurs after removal

_____ Crowds normal tissue

_____ Remains localized

6. Match each diagnostic laboratory test with the type of cancer it is used to detect.

Diagnostic Test	Type of Cancer Detected
_____ Serum calcitonin levels	a. Thyroid, breast, and oat (small) cell cancer in the lung
_____ Carcinoembryonic antigen	b. Gynecologic and pancreatic cancers
_____ PSA	c. Prostate cancer
_____ CA-125	d. Colorectal cancer

7. The complete blood cell profile of a patient diagnosed with cancer shows a reduction in the number of circulating platelets. Which term is used to describe this condition?
a. Leukopenia
b. Thrombocytopenia
c. Anemia
d. Neutropenia

8. Discuss the use of radiation treatments to manage cancer.

9. What is the mode of action for chemotherapy drugs?

10. Sometimes cancer is described as *metastatic*. What does this mean?

11. How does metastasis occur?

12. Use of the immune system to counteract the destruction of cancer cells is known as

    _____. _____ may be used to remove a tumor, lesion, and surrounding malignant tissue.

13. Indicate whether each statement is true or false.

    a. _____ Alopecia in patients undergoing chemotherapy results from damage to the hair follicle.

    b. _____ Alopecia is permanent.

    c. _____ Hair that regrows may be of a different color and/or texture than original hair.

14. List and discuss the complications involving the gastrointestinal system associated with the administration of chemotherapy.

15. Why is the patient with cancer at risk for developing nutritional problems?

16. For what nutritional disturbances is the patient with cancer at risk?

Exercise 2

Virtual Hospital Activity

30 minutes

- Sign in to work at Pacific View Regional Hospital for Period of Care 4. (*Note:* If you are already in the virtual hospital from a previous exercise, click **Leave the Floor** and then **Restart the Program** to get to the sign-in window.)
- Click **Chart** and then **405** to view Pablo Rodriguez's chart. (*Remember:* You are not able to visit patients or administer medications during Period of Care 4. You are only able to review patients records.)
- Click the **Nursing Admission** tab and review the information given.

1. What is Pablo Rodriguez's medical diagnosis?

2. According to the Nursing Admission, how does the patient describe his prognosis?

3. When was Pablo Rodriguez diagnosed with lung cancer?

• Click the **History and Physical** tab and review the reports.

4. How has Pablo Rodriguez's cancer been treated?

5. Does he have any family history of cancer?

6. Does his social history contain any risk factors for his diagnosis of lung cancer?

7. What psychosocial changes have resulted in his life because of the cancer?

8. Discuss the physical changes that have taken place as a result of Pablo Rodriguez's cancer.

9. Discuss Pablo Rodriguez's emotional readiness for death.

10. What emotional concerns have been voiced by the patient?

11. What therapeutic behaviors by the nurse are essential at this time?

12. What factors may put Pablo Rodriguez at risk for infection?

13. In addition to the nausea and vomiting, is Pablo Rodriguez suffering from any other complications of the gastrointestinal system?

14. Has Pablo Rodriguez experienced any nutritional disturbances during his illness?

LESSON **13**

Assessment of the Patient with Gastrointestinal Complications

Reading Assignment: Care of the Patient with a Gastrointestinal Disorder (Chapter 5)

Patient: Piya Jordan, Room 403

Objectives:

1. Identify clinical manifestations and causes of intestinal obstructions.
2. Develop nursing diagnoses appropriate for the patient experiencing an intestinal obstruction.
3. Explain operative measures used in cases of intestinal obstruction.
4. Identify common gastrointestinal disorders.
5. Identify tests used in the diagnosis of gastrointestinal disorders.
6. List medications used in the management of gastrointestinal disorders.

Exercise 1

Writing Activity

15 minutes

1. Describe the two types of intestinal obstructions.

   a. Mechanical obstruction:

   b. Nonmechanical obstruction:

2. The signs and symptoms associated with a bowel obstruction will be determined by the

   _____ and _____ of _____.

3. When caring for a patient suspected of having an intestinal obstruction, which manifestations would be considered early symptoms? Select all that apply.

   _____ Loud bowel sounds

   _____ High-pitched bowel sounds

   _____ Vomiting

   _____ Constipation

   _____ Absence of bowel sounds

   _____ Frequent bowel sounds

   _____ Abdominal pain

4. Identify several causes of mechanical intestinal obstructions.

5. Which are causes associated with nonmechanical intestinal obstructions? Select all that apply.

   _____ Complications from surgery

   _____ Bowel tumors

   _____ Electrolyte abnormalities

   _____ Thoracic spinal trauma

   _____ Lumbar spinal trauma

   _____ Embolism or atherosclerosis of the mesenteric arteries

   _____ Impacted feces

6. _____ Paralytic ileus is the most common type of nonmechanical intestinal obstruction. (True/False)

7. Which symptoms, if present, can be associated with a paralytic ileus? Select all that apply.

   _____ Increased abdominal girth

   _____ Distention

   _____ Urinary frequency

   _____ Elevated white blood cell count

   _____ Vomiting

8. Which interventions are done to reduce the risk for developing a paralytic ileus? Select all that apply.

   _____ Abdominal assessment

   _____ IV therapy

   _____ Maintenance of NG tube

   _____ Increase in patient activity

   _____ Deep breathing exercises

Exercise 2

Writing Activity

30 minutes

1. Match each diagnostic test with its correct description.

Diagnostic Test	**Description**
_____ Upper gastrointestinal study	a. Aspiration and review of stomach contents to determine acid production
_____ Tube gastric analysis	
_____ Esophagogastroduodenoscopy	b. Radiographs of the lower esophagus, stomach, and duodenum using barium sulfate as a contrast medium
_____ Lower GI endoscopy	c. Visualization of the upper GI tract by a flexible scope
_____ Bernstein test	d. An acid-perfusion test using hydrochloric acid
	e. Assessment of the lower GI tract with a scope

2. What is a KUB?

3. When providing education to a patient diagnosed with GERD, what information should be included in the teaching session? Select all that apply.

_____ Eat a low-fat, low-protein diet

_____ Avoid eating 4 to 6 hours before bedtime

_____ Remain upright for 1 to 2 hours after meals

_____ Avoid eating in bed

_____ Eat 4 to 6 small meals per day

_____ Reduce caffeine intake

4. Match each gastrointestinal disorder with its correct description.

Gastrointestinal Disorder

_____ GERD

_____ Candidiasis

_____ Gastritis

_____ Irritable bowel syndrome

_____ Ulcerative colitis

_____ Crohn's disease

_____ Diverticulosis

Description

a. The presence of pouchlike herniations through the muscular layers of the colon

b. Characterized by inflammation of segments of the GI tract, resulting in a cobblestone-like appearance of the mucosa

c. Episodic bowel dysfunction characterized by intestinal pain, disturbed defecation, or abdominal distention

d. The formation of tiny abscesses on mucosa and submucosa of the colon, producing drainage and sloughing of the mucosa and subsequent ulcerations

e. The backward flow of stomach acid into the esophagus

f. A fungal infection presenting as white patches on the mucous membranes

g. Inflammation of the lining of the stomach

5. Match each gastrointestinal medication with its correct classification.

Medication

_____ Maalox

_____ Pepcid

_____ Prevacid

_____ Carafate

_____ Cytotec

Classification

a. Proton pump inhibitor

b. Antacid

c. Antisecretory and cytoprotective agent

d. Mucosal healing agent

e. Histamine H_2 receptor blocker

6. Which alternative therapies may provide relief for excessive flatulence? Select all that apply.

_____ Comfrey

_____ Queen Anne's lace seeds

_____ Anise

_____ Chaparral

_____ Peppermint oil

_____ Spearmint extract

7. Gastrointestinal disorders may be more prevalent in certain ethnic groups. Which ethnic group has a higher incidence of inflammatory bowel disease?
   a. Caucasian
   b. African-American
   c. Asian-American
   d. Americans of Middle Eastern descent

8. The increased incidence of gastritis in older adults can be attributed to the decreased secretion of

   _____.

9. What is a colectomy? What is a colostomy?

Exercise 3

Virtual Hospital Activity

15 minutes

- Sign in to work at Pacific View Regional Hospital for Period of Care 1. (*Note:* If you are already in the virtual hospital from a previous exercise, click **Leave the Floor** and then **Restart the Program** to get to the sign-in window.)
- From the Patient List, select Piya Jordan (Room 403).
- Click **Get Report** and read the Clinical Report.
- Click **Go to Nurse's Station**.
- Click **Chart** and then **403** to view Piya Jordan's chart.
- Click the **Emergency Department** tab and review the information given.

1. What are Piya Jordan's primary complaints upon arrival to the emergency department?

2. What are Piya Jordan's vital signs at admission?

   HR:

   T:

   RR:

   BP:

3. What can Piya Jordan's hypotension most likely be attributed to?
   a. The presence of infection
   b. An elevation in blood glucose values
   c. Hypokalemia
   d. Dehydration

4. What diagnostic tests were ordered for Piya Jordan in the emergency department?

5. According to the ED physician's progress notes, what are the abnormal findings on the physical assessment that support a potential bowel obstruction?

6. What are the treatment goals of the care for a patient experiencing an intestinal obstruction?

7. Initial management of the patient's condition included the placement of an NG tube. The NG tube can serve a variety of functions. Match each function with its correct description.

Function	Description
_____ Decompression	a. Irrigation of the stomach, used in cases of active bleeding, poisoning, or gastric dilation
_____ Feeding	b. Removal of secretions and gases from the GI tract
_____ Compression	c. Internal application of pressure by means of an inflated balloon to prevent internal GI hemorrhage
_____ Lavage	d. Instillation of liquid supplements into the stomach

8. Piya Jordan has had the NG tube inserted for _____.

• Click **Surgical Reports** in the chart.

9. Piya Jordan has had a right hemicolectomy. Which description of the procedure is most accurate?
   a. Resection of ascending colon and hepatic flexure; ileum anastomosed to transverse colon
   b. Resection of the splenic flexure, descending colon, and sigmoid colon; transverse colon anastomosed to rectum
   c. Resection of part of the descending colon, the sigmoid colon, and upper rectum; descending colon anastomosed to remaining rectum
   d. Resection of the descending colon, the sigmoid colon, and upper rectum to the ileum and anastomosed to the transverse colon

• Click **Return to Nurses' Station**.
• Click **403** at the bottom the screen to go to Piya Jordan's room.
• Review the **Initial Observations**.

10. According to the Initial Observations, blood is being administered to Piya Jordan. What laboratory results will necessitate close observation to determine the effectiveness of this intervention?

11. What will the nurse need to monitor concerning the blood transfusion?

12. Piya Jordan has remained NPO since the surgery. What information will the nurse need to monitor to ensure she is adequately hydrated?

13. Which position will be most therapeutic to Piya Jordan in the postoperative period?
    a. Semi-Fowler's
    b. Fowler's
    c. Prone
    d. Side-lying

Colorectal Cancer and Care of the Patient After Gastrointestinal Surgery

Reading Assignment: Care of the Surgical Patient (Chapter 2)
Care of the Patient with a Gastrointestinal Disorder (Chapter 5)

Patient: Piya Jordan, Room 403

Objectives:

1. Identify risk factors associated with the development of colorectal cancer.
2. List the warning signs and symptoms associated with a diagnosis of colorectal cancer.
3. Identify the assessment priorities for the postoperative patient.
4. Discuss the safe use of narcotics administered in the postoperative period.
5. Discuss the potential for postoperative complications.

Exercise 1

Writing Activity

15 minutes

1. Indicate whether each statement is true or false.

   a. _____ Cancer of the colon and rectum is the second leading cause of cancer in the United States.

   b. _____ In the early stages, colorectal cancer is often asymptomatic.

2. What factors may be associated with colorectal? Select all that apply.

   _____ Ulcerative colitis

   _____ Peritonitis

   _____ Diverticulosis

   _____ Elevated bacterial counts in the colon

   _____ Vegan diets

   _____ High dietary fat intake

   _____ Dietary intake high in cruciferous vegetables

3. The nurse is caring for a patient who is 36 years old. She has a family history of colon cancer. What recommendations should be provided to this patient concerning screening?
   a. Begin colonoscopy screening after age 50.
   b. Have a baseline colonoscopy before age 50.
   c. Have an initial colonoscopy before age 40 and then every 5 years after.
   d. No special screening recommendations are needed.

4. Which symptoms are associated with the later stages of colorectal cancer? Select all that apply.

   _____ Constipation

   _____ Diarrhea

   _____ Abdominal pain

   _____ Anemia

   _____ Weakness

   _____ Emaciation

5. The incidence of colorectal cancer increases in persons over age _____.

6. The 5-year survival rate for early localized colorectal cancer is _____%; for cancer that has

   spread to adjacent organs and lymph nodes, it is _____%.

7. _____ refers to weakness and emaciation associated with general ill
   health and malnutrition.

8. What details should be included in the assessment of a surgical incision?

Exercise 2

Virtual Hospital Activity

30 minutes

- Sign in to work at Pacific View Regional Hospital for Period of Care 1. (*Note:* If you are already in the
  virtual hospital from a previous exercise, click **Leave the Floor** and then **Restart the Program** to get to
  the sign-in window.)
- From the Patient List, select Piya Jordan (Room 403).
- Click **Get Report** and read the Clinical Report.
- Click **Go to Nurses' Station** and then click the **Drug** icon. Find the entry for meperidine and review.

1. Based on your review of the shift report, which care factors appear to be of high priority?

2. The assessment findings of which of the patient's body systems demonstrate the potential for
   developing postoperative complications?
   a. Respiratory system
   b. Renal system
   c. Integumentary system
   d. Reproductive system

- Click **Return to Nurses' Station**.
- Click **403** and read the **Initial Observations**.
- Click **Take Vital Signs** and then on **Clinical Alerts** and review the information given.
- Click **Patient Care** and complete a head-to-toe assessment.

3. Discuss the proper assessment of bowel sounds for this patient.

4. What is the purpose of the Jackson-Pratt drain? How long will it need to be in place for Piya Jordan?

5. When the nurse is providing care for Piya Jordan, what should be monitored and recorded regarding the NG tube?

6. Piya Jordan has a reduced aeration to the left lower lobe. What interventions can promote improved aeration and a reduction in potential complications?

- Click **Chart** and then **403** to view Piya Jordan's chart.
- Click the **Nurse's Notes** tab and review the information given.

7. According to the Wednesday 0630 Nurse's Notes, Piya Jordan's meperidine PCA was discontinued because of suspicions of toxicity. Which clinical manifestations are associated with meperidine toxicity? Select all that apply.

_____ Respiratory depression

_____ Systolic hypertension

_____ Clammy skin

_____ Cyanosis

_____ Stupor

_____ Coma

_____ Diarrhea

8. In the event that pharmacologic intervention is needed to treat meperidine toxicity, which medication may be administered?
a. Compazine
b. Phenergan
c. Famotidine
d. Narcan

9. Which conditions may increase a patient's risk for meperidine toxicity? Select all that apply.

_____ Advancing age

_____ Diabetes

_____ Cardiovascular disorders

_____ Renal impairments

_____ Hypertension

- Click **Return to Room 403**.
- Click **Physical Assessment** and complete a head-to-toe assessment.

10. Which assessment findings for Piya Jordan are consistent with the suspected meperidine toxicity? Select all that apply.

   _____ Glasgow Coma Scale results

   _____ Confusion

   _____ Temperature 99.9

   _____ Respiratory rate 23

   _____ Slurred, slowed speech

   _____ Restless

- Click **Patient Care** and then **Nurse-Client Interactions**.
- Select and view the video titled **0735: Pain—Adverse Drug Event**. (*Note:* Check the virtual clock to see whether enough time has elapsed. You can use the fast-forward feature to advance the time by 2-minute intervals if the video is not yet available. Then click again on **Patient Care** and **Nurse-Client Interactions** to refresh the screen.)

11. What problems were encountered during the previous evening with regard to the use of the PCA pump?

12. What patient/family concerns during the video indicate the need for education?

13. What issues does the nurse need to address with Piya Jordan's daughter in particular?

Exercise 3

Virtual Hospital Activity

15 minutes

- Sign in to work at Pacific View Regional Hospital for Period of Care 3. (*Note:* If you are already in the virtual hospital from a previous exercise, click **Leave the Floor** and then **Restart the Program** to get to the sign-in window.)
- From the Patient List, select Piya Jordan (Room 403).
- Click **Get Report** and read the Clinical Report.
- Click **Go to Nurses' Station**.
- Click **403** at the bottom of the screen to enter the patient's room.
- Read the **Initial Observations**.

1. Have there been any changes in mental status since Period of Care 1?

2. What changes have been made to the type and/or administration of Piya Jordan's pain medication?

3. How does Piya Jordan rate her pain at this time?

- Click **Chart** and then **403** to view Piya Jordan's chart.
- Click the **Surgical Reports** tab and review the reports.

4. What type of surgery was planned for Piya Jordan? What surgical procedure was actually completed?

5. What are the most common complications associated with the surgery performed on Piya Jordan? Select all that apply.

_____ Hemorrhage

_____ Infection

_____ Blood loss

_____ Pneumonia

_____ Wound dehiscence

_____ Blood clots

_____ Paralytic ileus

6. What is Piya Jordan's postoperative diagnosis?

- Click the **Physician's Orders** tab and review the information given.

7. What medications and/or interventions have been ordered to assess and reduce the patient's postoperative risk of infection?

8. Which assessments will provide information to determine the presence of an infection? Select all that apply.

_____   Vital signs

_____   Appearance of urine in Foley catheter bag

_____   Abdominal incision

         Lung fields

_____   Patency of Jackson-Pratt drain

- Click **Return to Room 403**.
- Click **Take Vital Signs** and review the findings.
- Click **Patient Care** and perform a head-to-toe assessment.

9. Does Piya Jordan demonstrate any symptoms associated with a potential infection?

10. What interventions have been ordered to reduce the patient's risk for pulmonary complications?

Notes:

Notes:

Notes:

Notes:

Notes:

Notes:

Notes:

Notes:

Notes:

Notes: